The Ocular Circulation

The Ocular Circulation

Jeffrey W. Kiel, Ph.D.

www.morganclaypool.com

ISBN: 9781615041688   paperback
ISBN: 9781615041695   ebook

DOI 10.4199/C00024ED1V01Y201012ISP012

A Publication in the Morgan & Claypool Publishers series
SYNTHESIS LECTURES ON INTEGRATED SYSTEMS PHYSIOLOGY:
FROM MOLECULE TO FUNCTION TO DISEASE

Lecture #11
Series Editor: D. Neil Granger, *Louisiana State University Health Sciences Center*
                        Joey P. Granger, *University of Mississippi Medical Center*
Series ISSN
Synthesis Lectures on Integrated Systems Physiology: From Molecule to Function to Disease
Print 1947-945X   Electronic 1947-9468

Synthesis Lectures on Integrated Systems Physiology: From Molecule to Function to Disease

Editors
D. Neil Granger, *Louisiana State University Health Sciences Center*
Joey P. Granger, *University of Mississippi Medical Center*

Physiology is a scientific discipline devoted to understanding the functions of the body. It addresses function at multiple levels, including molecular, cellular, organ, and system. An appreciation of the processes that occur at each level is necessary to understand function in health and the dysfunction associated with disease. Homeostasis and integration are fundamental principles of physiology that account for the relative constancy of organ processes and bodily function even in the face of substantial environmental changes. This constancy results from integrative, cooperative interactions of chemical and electrical signaling processes within and between cells, organs and systems. This eBook series on the broad field of physiology covers the major organ systems from an integrative perspective that addresses the molecular and cellular processes that contribute to homeostasis. Material on pathophysiology is also included throughout the eBooks. The state-of the art treatises were produced by leading experts in the field of physiology. Each eBook includes stand-alone information and is intended to be of value to students, scientists, and clinicians in the biomedical sciences. Since physiological concepts are an ever-changing work-in-progress, each contributor will have the opportunity to make periodic updates of the covered material.

The Ocular Circulation
Jeffrey W. Kiel, Ph.D.
2010

Colonic Motility: From Bench Side to Bedside
Sushil K. Sarna
2010

Angiogenesis
Thomas H. Adair, Jean-Pierre Montani
2010

Vascular Biology of the Placenta
Yuping Wang
2010

The Ocular Circulation

Jeffrey W. Kiel, Ph.D.
University of Texas Health Science Center at San Antonio

SYNTHESIS LECTURES ON INTEGRATED SYSTEMS PHYSIOLOGY: FROM MOLECULE TO FUNCTION TO DISEASE #11

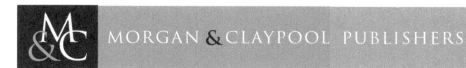

MORGAN & CLAYPOOL PUBLISHERS

ABSTRACT

This presentation describes the unique anatomy and physiology of the vascular beds that serve the eye. The needs for an unobstructed light path from the cornea to the retina and a relatively fixed corneal curvature and distance between refractive structures pose significant challenges for the vasculature to provide nutrients and remove metabolic waste. To meet these needs, the ocular vascular beds are confined to the periphery of the posterior two thirds of the eye and a surrogate circulation provides a continuous flow of aqueous humor to nourish the avascular cornea, lens and vitreous compartment. The production of aqueous humor (and its ease of egress from the eye) also generates the intraocular pressure (IOP), which maintains the shape of the eye. However, the IOP also exerts a compressing force on the ocular blood vessels that is higher than elsewhere in the body. This is particularly true for the intraocular veins, which must have a pressure higher than IOP to remain patent, and so the IOP is the effective venous pressure for the intraocular vascular beds. Consequently, the ocular circulation operates at a lower perfusion pressure gradient than elsewhere in the body and is more at risk for ischemic damage when faced with low arterial pressure, particularly if IOP is elevated. This risk and the specialized tissues of the eye give rise to the fascinating physiology of the ocular circulations.

KEYWORDS

ocular circulation, choroid, intraocular pressure, aqueous dynamics, local control, autoregulation

Contents

x

Acknowledgments

The author's work cited in this presentation was supported by the Texas Affiliate of the American Heart Association, the National Institutes of Health, the Lions Club International, Research to Prevent Blindness, and the van Heuven endowment. The assistance of Ms. Alma Maldonado is gratefully acknowledged.

Jeffrey W. Kiel, Ph.D.
December 2010

CHAPTER 1

Introduction

The ocular circulation is an interesting example of vascular adaptation in the service of organ function. A spherical shape, a precise corneal curvature and distance between refractive structures and the photoreceptors, and a clear path for light transmission are structural design features of the mammalian visual organ. Those structural features pose significant challenges for the vasculature to provide nutrients and remove metabolic waste. To meet these needs, the ocular vascular beds are confined to the periphery of the posterior segment and a surrogate circulation provides a continuous flow of aqueous humor to nourish the avascular cornea, lens and vitreous compartment. The production of aqueous humor (and its ease of egress from the eye) also generates the intraocular pressure (IOP), which maintains the shape of the eye. However, the IOP also exerts a compressing force on the ocular blood vessels that is higher than found typically in other organs or tissues. This is particularly true for the intraocular veins, which must have a pressure higher than IOP to remain patent, and so the IOP is the effective venous pressure for the intraocular vascular beds. Consequently, the ocular circulation operates at a lower perfusion pressure gradient than elsewhere in the body and is more at risk for ischemic damage when faced with low arterial pressure, particularly if IOP is elevated.

CHAPTER 2

Anatomy

2.1 GENERAL EYE FEATURES

The outer coats of the eye are the cornea and sclera; their juncture is the limbus (Fig 2.1). The interior of the eye is divided into the anterior and posterior segments. The anterior segment includes the cornea, iris, ciliary body and lens as well as the spaces of the anterior and posterior chambers filled with aqueous humor. The posterior segment includes the retina, choroid and optic nerve head as well as the vitreous compartment filled with vitreous humor.

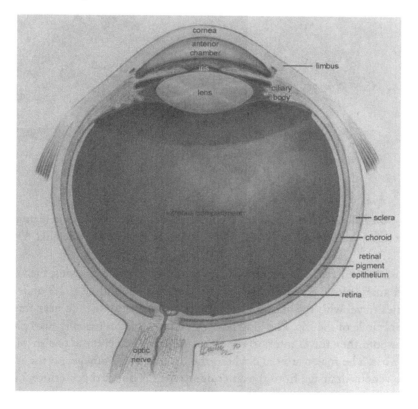

Figure 2.1: Illustration of the human eye. Reproduced with permission from NEI-NIH `ftp://ftp.nei.nih.gov/eyean/eye12-72.tif`

2.2   VASCULAR SUPPLY AND DRAINAGE

The arterial input to the eye is provided by several branches from the ophthalmic artery, which is derived from the internal carotid artery in most mammals (Fig 2.2, left). These branches include the central retinal artery, the short and long posterior ciliary arteries, and the anterior ciliary arteries. Venous outflow from the eye is primarily via the vortex veins and the central retinal vein, which merge with the superior and inferior ophthalmic veins that drain into the cavernous sinus, the pterygoid venous plexus and the facial vein (Fig 2.2, right). In some species (e.g., rodents and lagomorphs), the orbital veins form a sinus.

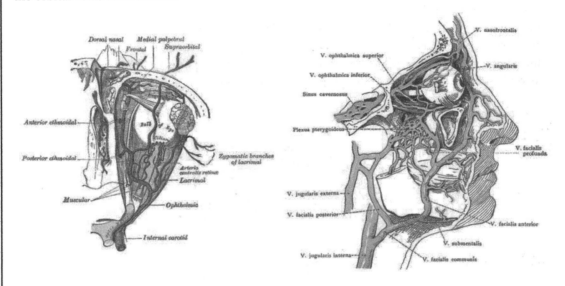

Figure 2.2: Arterial (left) and venous (right) connections to the systemic circulation. Reproduced from *Anatomy of the Human Body,* Gray, H., 2th Edition, Lea & Febiger, Philadelphia, 1954.

The iris and ciliary body are supplied by the anterior ciliary arteries, the long posterior ciliary arteries and anatosmotic connections from the anterior choroid (Fig 2.3 and 2.4). The anterior ciliary arteries travel with the extraocular muscles and pierce the sclera near the limbus to join the major arterial circle of the iris. The long posterior ciliary arteries (usually two) pierce the sclera near the posterior pole, then travel anteriorly between the sclera and choroid to also join the major arterial circle of the iris. The major arterial circle of the iris gives off branches to the iris and ciliary body. Most of the venous drainage from the anterior segment is directed posteriorly into the choroid and thence into the vortex veins.

The retina is supplied by the central retinal artery and the short posterior ciliary arteries (Fig 2.3). The central retinal artery travels in or beside the optic nerve as it pierces the sclera then branches to supply the layers of the inner retina (i.e., the layers closest to the vitreous compartment).

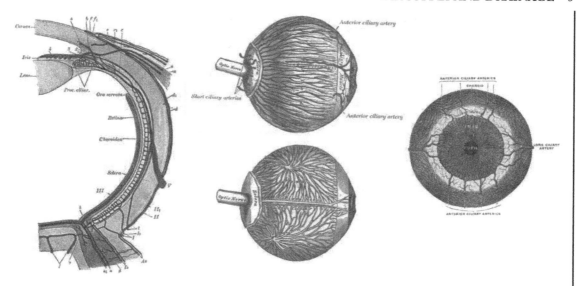

Figure 2.3: Diagrams of the blood vessels of the eye. Course of vasa centralia retinæ: α. Arteria. α_l. Vena centralis retinæ. β. Anastomosis with vessels of outer coats. γ. Anastomosis with branches of short posterior ciliary arteries. δ. Anastomosis with chorioideal vessels. Course of vasa ciliar. postic. brev.: I. Arteriæ, and I$_l$. Venæ ciliar. postic. brev. II. Episcleral artery. II$_l$. Episcleral vein. III. Capillaries of lamina choriocapillaris. Course of vasa ciliar. postic. long.: 1. ciliar. post. longa. 2. Circulus iridis major cut across. 3. Branches to ciliary body. 4. Branches to iris. Course of vasa ciliar. ant.: d. Arteria. d$_l$. Vena ciliar. ant. b. Junction with the circulus iridis major. c. Junction with lamina choriocapill. e. Arterial, and e$_l$. Venous episcleral branches. d. Arterial, and d$_l$. Venous branches to conjunctiva scleræ. f. Arterial, and f$_l$. Venous branches to corneal border. V. Vena vorticosa. S. Transverse section of sinus venosus scleræ. Reproduced from *Anatomy of the Human Body,* Gray, H., 2th Edition, Lea & Febiger, Philadelphia, 1954.

There are marked species differences in the inner retinal vascularization, with primates having a complex 4-zone arrangement and an avascular zone at the fovea, lagomorphs having a rather simple narrow band of superficial vessels, rodents having a wagon-wheel spoke-like arrangement and guinea pigs having no inner retinal vessels (Fig 2.5 and 2.6). Retinal venules and veins coalesce into the central retinal vein, which exits the eye with the optic nerve parallel and counter-current to the central retinal artery.

The short posterior ciliary arteries (typically 6-12) pierce the sclera around the optic nerve then arborize to form the arterioles of the dense outer layer of conduit vessels of the choroid (Fig 2.3, 2.4, 2.7). The arterioles the give off roughly perpendicular terminal arterioles that supply lobules of choriocapillaries that comprise the sheet-like layer of the choriocapillaris adjacent to Bruch's membrane, the retinal pigment and the outer segments of the photoreceptors (Fig 2.7). The chorio-

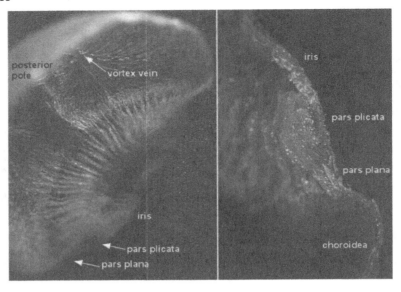

Figure 2.4: Bisected vascular cast of the rabbit eye (left) and rabbit anterior segment[1]. Reproduced with permission from Investigative Ophthalmology & Visual Science.

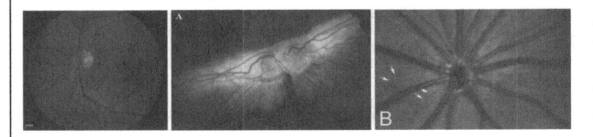

Figure 2.5: Fundus photographs of the human (left), rabbit (middle) and rat (right) retina.[2,3]. Reproduced with permission from Investigative Ophthalmology & Visual Science[1]. Reproduced with permission from American Physiological Society and Investigative Ophthalmology & Visual Science[2,3].

capillaris lobules drain into venules that join the larger venules of the outer conduit layer that coalesce into the 4-5 vortex veins that pierce the sclera at the equator.

The vascular supply of the optic nerve is complex (Fig 2.8). The optic nerve has three zones referenced to the lamina cribosa, the connective tissue extension of the sclera through which the optic nerve axons and the central retinal artery and vein pass. The prelaminar (i.e., inside the eye relative to the lamina cribosa) optic nerve is supplied by collaterals from the choroid and retina circulations.

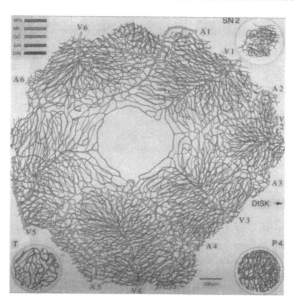

Figure 2.6: Primate foveal avascular zone[4]. Reproduced with permission from Society for Neuroscience.

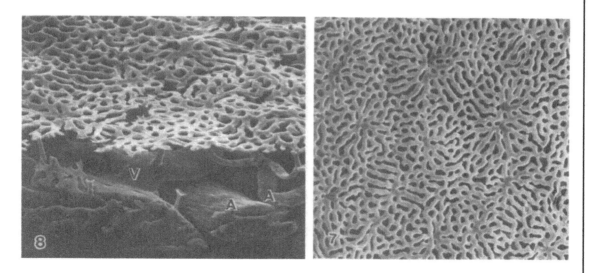

Figure 2.7: Vascular casts of the cat choroid showing arrangement of conduit vessels to choriocapillaris (left) and sheet-like structure of choriocapillaris viewed from the retina (right)[5]. Reproduced with permission from Investigative Ophthalmology & Visual Science.

The laminar zone is supplied by branches from the short posterior ciliary and pial arteries. The post laminar zone is supplied by the pial arteries. Venous drainage is via the central retinal vein and pial veins. For the optic nerve vessels, the laminar zone marks the transition from exposure to the IOP to the cerebral fluid pressure within the optic nerve sheath.

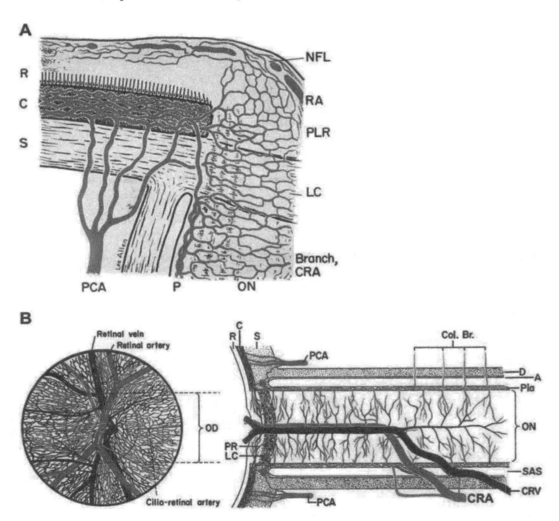

Figure 2.8: Schematic of optic nerve circulation[6]. Reproduced with permission from Progress in Retinal and Eye Research, Elsevier.

2.3   INNERVATION

Autonomic innervation of the ocular circulations is restricted to the vessels of the uvea (i.e., the choroid, ciliary body and iris) and optic nerve; the retina appears to lack sympathetic and parasympathetic nerves[7-9]. The postganglionic sympathetic nerves originate in the superior cervical ganglion. Parasympathetic innervation originates in the pterygopalatine ganglion via the facial nerve. In the choroid of primates and some species of birds, a network of ganglion cells has been identified similar to the enteric nervous system of the gut, but their functional significance is unclear[10,11].

CHAPTER 3

Blood flow measuring techniques

Although the blood vessels of the iris and inner retina are tantalizingly observable through the clear cornea, blood flow measurement in the eye is extremely difficult. Conspiring against simple approaches are the inaccessible locations of the arterial inputs and venous outputs within the bony orbit, the complex intermixing of the different vascular beds and the need to preserve the normal IOP. What follows is a brief description of some of the more common ocular blood flow measuring techniques.

The normally clear optical path from cornea-to-retina lends itself to optical imaging techniques. The earliest of these was film-based (now digital) fundus photography, which evolved into scanning laser ophthalmoscopy and optical coherence tomography. A digital video-based device, the retinal vessel analyzer (Imedos, Jena, Germany), is an imaging variant specific for measuring retinal vessel diameters. All can provide information about retinal vessel caliber responses to perturbations or drugs; however, a measurement of blood velocity in the same vessel is needed to calculate volumetric blood flow. Such velocity measurements in larger retinal vessels are typically done with a separate, dual-beam laser Doppler velocimeter. (A device, the Canon Laser Blood Flowmeter, combining retinal vessel diameter and blood velocity measurement in one instrument was briefly available commercially, but few were made or sold.)

Fundus imaging also gave rise to fluorescein and indocyanine green angiography to track dye movement through the vessels of the inner retina and choroid, respectively. High frequency angiograms provide information about regional blood velocity or transit time rather than volumetric blood flow. Two other methods that provide velocity information are the laser Doppler speckle technique used for the retinal and optic nerve head microcirculations, and ultrasound color Doppler imaging used for the ophthalmic artery, the central retinal artery and the short posterior ciliary arteries.

Laser Doppler flowmetry provides a measurement of red blood cell flux (i.e., the product of mean velocity and the number of moving cells) in a small volume of laser-illuminated tissue. Both fundus camera and fiber optic-based units are used; fundus camera units are used primarily for the optic nerve head and sub-foveal choroid, and fiber optic units are used primarily for intravitreal probe measurements of the choroid in animals with few retinal vessels or transcleral ciliary body and choroid measurements. Laser Doppler flowmetry (LDF) has the advantage of providing continuous measurements. However, it does not provide volumetric flow measurements and so measurements at different sites or between subjects are difficult to compare; LDF is much better suited for recording site-specific responses to perturbations.

For many years, the primary technique for animal ocular blood flow measurements was the radioactive (now colored) microsphere technique. The technique requires injection of the microspheres (originally 15 micron diameter spheres) into the left ventricle followed by quantification of the number of spheres trapped in the tissue of interest relative to an arterial blood sample taken at a known rate during the injection. The intraventricular injection is invasive and the technique requires death of the animal to harvest the tissue, but it does provide a quantitative measurement of tissue blood flow at the time of injection.

Some of the other less common ocular blood flow measuring techniques include scleral heat clearance, antipyrine autoradiography, pulsatile ocular blood flow (derived from the cardiac synchronous fluctuations in intraocular pressure or the cornea-to-retina distance), magnetic resonance imaging and Doppler optical coherence tomography.

CHAPTER 4

Ocular perfusion pressure, IOP and the ocular Starling resistor effect

The pressure gradient from arterial input to venous output and the resistance imparted by the fluid composition and vascular geometry determine blood flow through a vessel or tissue. In the eye, the pressure gradients begin with the pressure in the supply arteries, i.e., the central retinal artery, the short posterior ciliary arteries, the long posterior ciliary arteries and the anterior ciliary arteries) and end with the venous pressures in the exiting veins (i.e., the central retinal vein and the vortex veins primarily). The resistance is set by the blood, and the net length, branching pattern and cross-sectional area of the specific circulation. In the eye, as elsewhere in the body, the pressure drop from the large supply arteries to the capillaries indicates that the primary site of resistance resides in the small arteries and arterioles. However, unlike most tissues, the intraocular veins experience a significant compressing force, the intraocular pressure (IOP), and so they act like Starling resistors, i.e., the pressure in the veins just before they exit the eye must exceed the IOP or they collapse (Fig 2.1)[12–16]. Consequently, the effective venous pressure for the ocular circulations is the IOP. For this reason, the ocular perfusion pressure (OPP) is defined as the mean arterial pressure (MAP, at eye level) minus the IOP. From this definition, it follows that raising the IOP while holding MAP constant at different levels should produce a family of pressure-flow curves, each going to zero when the IOP equals MAP, and these separate curves should resolve into a single curve when flow is plotted as a function of OPP. This behavior has been demonstrated in the rabbit choroid (Fig 2.2) and is assumed to be qualitatively similar in the other ocular circulations across species[17].

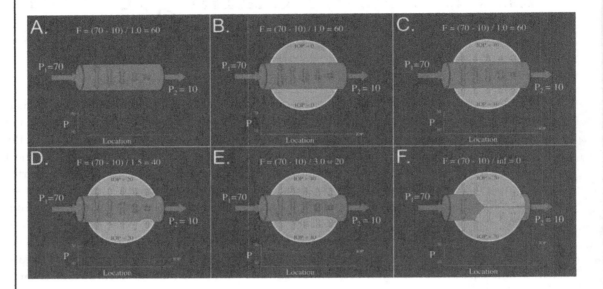

Figure 4.1: Ocular Starling resistor. A. Vessel flow (F) is a function of the pressure gradient (P1 – P2) along the vessel divided by the resistance. B - C. If the vessel passes through an organ (e.g., the eye) with a low tissue pressure (e.g., IOP), the pressure inside the vessel exceeds the pressure outside the vessel (i.e., the transmural pressure gradient) and so the vessel remains distended. D - E. If the tissue pressure is somewhat higher and exceeds the pressure at the lowest point inside the vessel (i.e., at the "venous" end), that region of the vessel will begin to collapse, which will increase the resistance to flow in that segment thereby raising the intravessel pressure until the transmural pressure is again slightly positive. F. If the tissue pressure becomes greater than the arterial input pressure, the vessel will collapse completely, the resistance will be infinite, and flow through the vessel will cease.

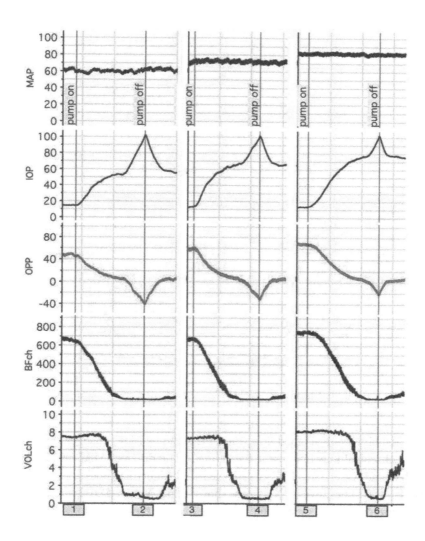

Figure 4.2: Effect of IOP on an ocular circulation. Traces are rabbit choroidal (primarily choriocapillaris) blood flow (BFch) and blood volume (VOLch) responses to increasing IOP by intraocular saline infusion at 30 μl/min as mean arterial pressure (MAP) is held constant at $\approx$60, 70 and 80 mmHg. Blood flow ceases and blood is expelled (i.e., the vessels collapse) when the IOP reaches the MAP and the ocular perfusion pressure (OPP) goes to zero. When the infusion is halted, the IOP declines until the OPP is again greater than zero whereupon the blood flow resumes and begins refilling the vessels. (Author's unpublished observations using LDF.).

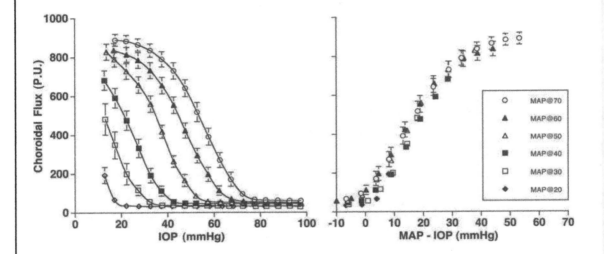

Figure 4.3: Rabbit choroidal blood flow (Flux, measured by LDF) changes with IOP and OPP (MAP – IOP). Left: choroidal Flux response to increasing IOP at different MAPs. Choroidal Flux falls as IOP nears the MAP and ceases when IOP exceeds the MAP. Right: the same data with choroidal Flux plotted against MAP - IOP. The curves superimpose showing that MAP – IOP is the effective ocular perfusion pressure[17]. Reproduced with permission from Investigative Ophthalmology & Visual Science.

CHAPTER 5

Ocular blood flow effects on IOP

Two conceptual models serve as the basis for understanding IOP (Fig 5.1). One model treats the IOP in terms of the ocular pressure-volume relation, which is an exponential function of the total ocular volume and the elasticity of the corneoscleral coat. This model is the theoretical basis for indentation tonometry and tonography[18,19]. The other model treats the steady-state IOP as a function of aqueous flow and outflow resistance[20]. This model is the theoretical basis for understanding ocular hypertension and hypotony as well as current drug and surgical treatment of ocular hypertension (i.e., elevated IOP). Both models provide insight into IOP physiology.

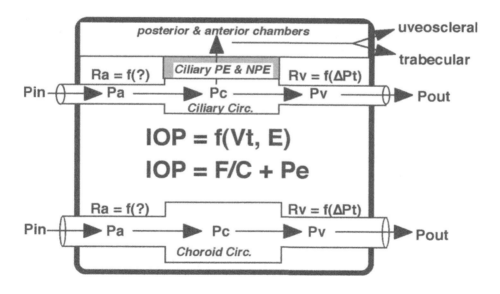

Figure 5.1: Schematic of IOP generation. (Pin: extraocular arterial pressure; Pa: intraocular arterial pressure; Pc: intraocular capillary pressure; Pv: intraocular venous pressure; Pout: extraocular venous pressure; Ra; arterial resistance; Rv: venous resistance; ΔPt: transmural pressure gradient; PE: pigment epithelium; NPE: nonpigment epithelium; Vt: total ocular volume; E: elastance or "rigidity" of the ocular coats; F: aqueous flow; C: outflow conductance or "facility"; Pe: episcleral venous pressure)[21]. Ciliary and choroidal Ra both designated with question marks to reflect ill-defined nature of neurohumoral and local control meachanisms involved[21]. Permission pending.

If the corneoscleral elastance is constant, changes in IOP must involve changes in ocular volume. The main contributors to the total ocular volume are the vitreous, lens, aqueous and blood. The volumes of the vitreous and lens are relatively stable and do not typically have an acute influence on IOP. The volumes of blood and aqueous are more labile and cause most variations in IOP. Changes in the volume of aqueous occur with transient imbalances in aqueous production and outflow. Similarly, ocular blood volume changes happen during transient imbalances in the flow of blood into and out of the eye. Most of the ocular blood volume is in the choroid, the highly vascularized tissue between the retina and sclera.

Because most IOP measurement techniques are discontinuous, the effect of blood flow (or more specifically, blood volume) on IOP generally goes unnoticed. However, continuous IOP measurement by direct cannulation shows that ocular blood volume contributes to IOP (Fig 5.2, top). For example, blood pressure synchronous changes in IOP are clearly evident. The IOP pulse is caused by pulsatile arterial inflow and steady venous outflow giving rise to fluctuations in ocular blood volume (Fig 5.2, bottom). This IOP pulse is used to estimate the pulsatile component of ocular blood flow[22].

Another example of the blood volume contribution to IOP is seen at death (Fig 5.3). If the heart is stopped quickly, the arterial pressure falls toward the mean circulatory filling pressure[23], blood flow into the eye stops and the residual blood volume drains out of the eye, resulting in a rapid net decrease in blood volume and an equally rapid fall in IOP. In anesthetized rabbits under control conditions, the IOP immediately before and after death are typically 15 mmHg and 7 mmHg, respectively. This occurs in seconds, which is too fast for aqueous dynamics to play a role in the IOP decrease.

In contrast to death, ocular blood volume is normally relatively well regulated during changes in arterial pressure[24]. As shown in Figure 5.4 (left), an acute increase in arterial pressure induced by occluding the aorta causes only a small increase in IOP due to choroidal vasoconstriction under control conditions. Both autoregulatory myogenic[24] and autonomic neural mechanisms[25] have been proposed to explain this response (see below). However, what is important to note is that when this choroidal regulation is abolished with a systemic vasodilator, a similar acute elevation of arterial pressure can elicit a significantly larger increase in IOP (Fig 5.4 right). Here again, it is clear that ocular blood volume contributes to total ocular volume and so influences the IOP.

A sustained pressure-induced increase in ocular blood volume does not produce a sustained increase in IOP as shown in Figure 5.5. Instead, the elevated IOP increases the pressure gradient for aqueous outflow, which causes a compensatory decrease of aqueous volume so that IOP gradually returns to baseline[24]. If the increase in blood volume is small, the compensation is relatively quick, whereas compensation for a larger increase in blood volume, as occurs when choroidal regulation is impaired, takes longer. In either situation, IOP falls below baseline when the arterial pressure-induced distention of the vasculature is abruptly ended, reflecting the compensatory loss of aqueous volume, which is gradually restored by continued aqueous production, which returns IOP to baseline. Such compensatory volume shifts were noted by Duke-Elder, who observed a marked shallowing

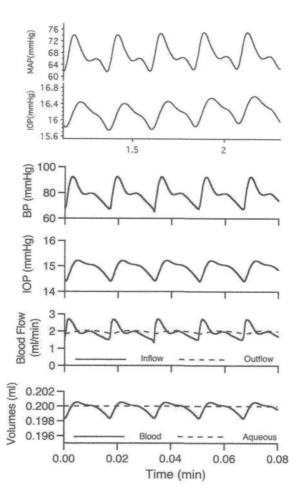

Figure 5.2: Top: Blood pressure and IOP recorded by direct cannulation of the central ear artery and vitreous compartment in an anesthetized rabbit. Bottom: Computer simulation showing cardiac synchronous IOP pulsations due to fluctuations in blood volume caused by pulsatile inflow of blood and steady outflow[21]. Permission pending.

of the anterior chamber and rise of IOP to 80 − 90 mmHg upon ligation of the vortex veins in anesthetized dogs, the most extreme method to cause choroidal engorgement[26].

The effect of blood volume on IOP is also apparent in the ocular pressure-volume relationship. In anesthetized rabbits, cumulative intraocular saline injections give different pressure-volume relationships when arterial pressure is held at different levels, which are all different from that ob-

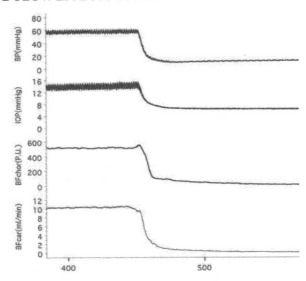

Figure 5.3: Drop in IOP occurs immediately upon cardiac arrest induced with an overdose of pentobarbital (100 mg/kg, i.v.) in a deeply anesthetized rabbit. Continued venous outflow without corresponding arterial inflow results in the net loss of blood volume responsible for the fall in IOP (BP: blood pressure; BFchor: choroidal blood flow by LDF; BFcar: carotid blood flow by transit-time ultrasound. Time in seconds.).

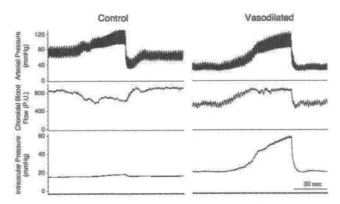

Figure 5.4: IOP responses to acute increases in arterial pressure in an anesthetized rabbit. Raising arterial pressure to 110 mmHg elicits a modest increase in IOP under control conditions (left) and a much larger increase when choroidal regulation is impaired by systemic vasodilation with hydralazine (right). The vasodilated IOP response is the largest recorded by the author[24]. Reproduced with permission from Experimental Eye Research, Elsevier.

[80] Schmetterer L, Findl O, Strenn K, et al. Role of NO in the O2 and CO2 responsiveness of cerebral and ocular circulation in humans *Am J Physiol.* 1997; 273: R2005–2012. 41

[81] Roth S. Post-ischemic hyperemia in the cat retina: the effects of adenosine receptor blockade *Curr Eye Res.* 1995; 14: 323–328. DOI: 10.3109/02713689509033533 41, 48, 50

[82] Bill A, Linder M, Linder J. The protective role of ocular sympathetic vasomotor nerves in acute arterial hypertension *Bibl. anat.* 1977; 16: 30 - 35. 42, 55

[83] Parver LM, Auker C, Carpenter DO. Choroidal blood flow as a heat dissipating mechanism in the macula *Am J Ophthal.* 1980; 89: 641 - 646. 43

[84] Nielsen B., Savard G., Richter E. A., Hargreaves M., Saltin B. Muscle blood flow and muscle metabolism during exercise and heat stress *J Appl Physiol.* 1990; 69: 1040–6. 43

[85] Parver LM, Auker CR, Carpenter DO, Doyle T. Choroidal blood flow II. reflexive control in the monkey *Arch. Ophthalmol.* 1982; 100: 1327–1330. 44

[86] Chemtob S, Beharry K, Rex J, et al. Ibuprofen enhances retinal and choroidal blood flow autoregulation in newborn piglets *Invest Ophthalmol Vis Sci.* 1991; 32: 1799 - 1807. 46

[87] Tamaki Y., Araie M., Kawamoto E., Eguchi S., Fujii H. Noncontact, two-dimensional measurement of retinal microcirculation using laser speckle phenomenon *Invest Ophthalmol Vis Sci.* 1994; 35: 3825–34.

[88] Harino S., Nishimura K., Kitanishi K., Suzuki M., Reinach P. Role of nitric oxide in mediating retinal blood flow regulation in cats *J Ocul Pharmacol Ther.* 1999; 15: 295–303. DOI: 10.1089/jop.1999.15.295 46

[89] Zuckerman R., Weiter J. J. Oxygen transport in the bullfrog retina *Exp Eye Res.* 1980; 30: 117–27. DOI: 10.1016/0014-4835(80)90106-2 47

[90] Linsenmeier R. A., Steinberg R. H. Effects of hypoxia on potassium homeostasis and pigment epithelial cells in the cat retina *J Gen Physiol.* 1984; 84: 945–70. DOI: 10.1085/jgp.84.6.945 47

[91] Linsenmeier R. A. Effects of light and darkness on oxygen distribution and consumption in the cat retina *J Gen Physiol.* 1986; 88: 521–42. DOI: 10.1085/jgp.88.4.521 47

[92] Birol G., Wang S., Budzynski E., Wangsa-Wirawan N. D., Linsenmeier R. A. Oxygen distribution and consumption in the macaque retina *Am J Physiol Heart Circ Physiol.* 2007; 293: H1696–704. DOI: 10.1152/ajpheart.00221.2007 47

[93] Bill A, Sperber GO. Control of retinal and choroidal blood flow *Eye.* 1990; 4: 319 - 325. 47, 48

[94] Shakoor A., Blair N. P., Mori M., Shahidi M. Chorioretinal vascular oxygen tension changes in response to light flicker *Invest Ophthalmol Vis Sci.* 2006; 47: 4962–5. DOI: 10.1167/iovs.06-0291

[95] Kiryu J, Asrani S, Shahidi M, Mori M, Zeimer R. Local Response of the Primate Retinal Microcirculation to Increased Metabolic Demand Induced by Flicker *Invest Ophthalmol Vis Sci.* 1995; 36: 1240–1246. 48

[96] Nagaoka T., Sakamoto T., Mori F., Sato E., Yoshida A. The effect of nitric oxide on retinal blood flow during hypoxia in cats *Invest Ophthalmol Vis Sci.* 2002; 43: 3037–44. 48, 49

[97] Sato E., Sakamoto T., Nagaoka T., et al. Role of nitric oxide in regulation of retinal blood flow during hypercapnia in cats *Invest Ophthalmol Vis Sci.* 2003; 44: 4947–53. DOI: 10.1167/iovs.03-0284 48

[98] Izumi N., Nagaoka T., Sato E., et al. Role of nitric oxide in regulation of retinal blood flow in response to hyperoxia in cats *Invest Ophthalmol Vis Sci.* 2008; 49: 4595–603. DOI: 10.1167/iovs.07-1667 48

[99] Stefansson E., Wagner H. G., Seida M. Retinal blood flow and its autoregulation measured by intraocular hydrogen clearance *Exp Eye Res.* 1988; 47: 669–78. DOI: 10.1016/0014-4835(88)90034-6 48, 49

[100] Kiel J. W., Hollingsworth M., Rao R., Chen M., Reitsamer H. A. Ciliary blood flow and aqueous humor production *Prog Retin Eye Res.* 52

[101] Chamot S. R., Movaffaghy A., Petrig B. L., Riva C. E. Iris blood flow response to acute decreases in ocular perfusion pressure: a laser Doppler flowmetry study in humans *Exp Eye Res.* 2000; 70: 107–12. DOI: 10.1006/exer.1999.0759 53

[102] Tomidokoro A., Araie M., Tamaki Y., Tomita K. In vivo measurement of iridial circulation using laser speckle phenomenon *Invest Ophthalmol Vis Sci.* 1998; 39: 364–71. 53

[103] Granstam E., Nilsson S. F. Non-adrenergic sympathetic vasoconstriction in the eye and some other facial tissues in the rabbit *Eur J Pharmacol.* 1990; 175: 175–86. DOI: 10.1016/0014-2999(90)90228-X 55, 57

[104] Zagvazdin Y, Fitzgerald MEC, Reiner A. Role of muscarinic cholinergic transmission in Edinger-Westphal nucleus-induced choroidal vasodilation in pigeon *Exp Eye Res.* 2000; 70: 315–27. DOI: 10.1006/exer.1999.0791 58

[105] Nilsson S. F., Linder J., Bill A. Characteristics of uveal vasodilation produced by facial nerve stimulation in monkeys, cats and rabbits *Exp Eye Res.* 1985; 40: 841–52. DOI: 10.1016/0014-4835(85)90129-0 58

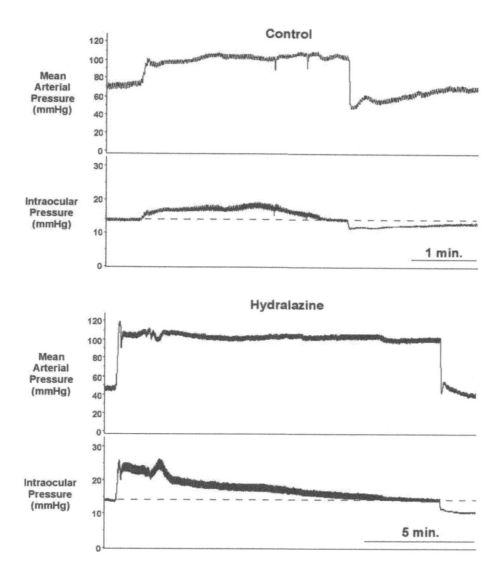

Figure 5.5: IOP responses to sustained increases in arterial pressure under control and vasodilated conditions in anesthetized rabbits. Raising arterial pressure mechanically to 110 mmHg under control conditions elicits a relatively small increase in IOP that returns to baseline relatively quickly; raising arterial pressure to the same level under vasodilated conditions results in a larger increase in IOP that takes longer to return to baseline. Restoration of baseline arterial pressure ends vascular engorgement and the undershoot of IOP reveals the compensatory loss of aqueous volume that returned IOP to baseline during the arterial pressure elevation[24]. Reproduced with permission from Experimental Eye Research, Elsevier.

tained post mortem (Fig 5.6)[27]. The original Friedenwald tables used in tonometry and tonography were based on enucleated eyes re-inflated with saline to achieve a normal IOP[19,28]. This procedure eliminated any blood volume buffering of the IOP response to additional saline injections. However, as Figure 5.6 shows, the pressure volume relationship and the ocular rigidity coefficient (an index of corneoscleral elastance) are both dependant on the arterial pressure distending the ocular vessels.

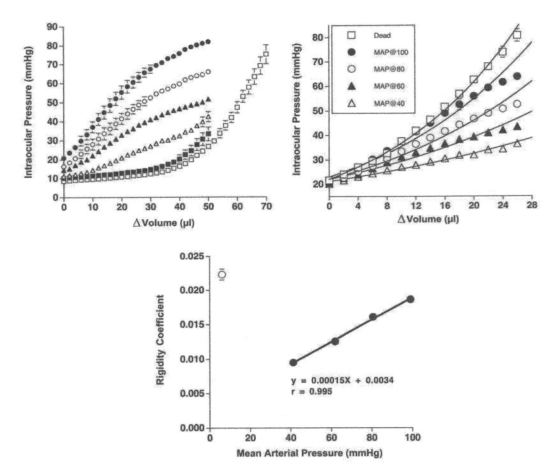

Figure 5.6: Effect of mean arterial pressure (MAP) on the intraocular pressure-volume relationship and ocular rigidity in anesthetized rabbits[27]. Reproduced with permission from Experimental Eye Research, Elsevier.

CHAPTER 6

Local control of ocular blood flow

The "local control" mechanisms operating in the ocular circulations are difficult to define. Based on more accessible circulations in other tissues, probable local control mechanisms in the eye include vascular responses linked to nearby tissue metabolism (e.g., reactive hyperemia, functional hyperemia and autoregulation), transmural pressure (e.g., myogenic response, reactive hyperemia and autoregulation), shear stress (flow-dependent vasodilation) and intercellular conduction. The relative roles of these mechanisms are difficult to define because the eye's complex vascular organization makes discrete perturbations that elicit unambiguous responses characteristic of a particular mechanism in a single vascular bed hard to achieve. Eliminating confounding neurohumoral inputs is an additional challenge. Consequently, it is often possible to infer that a response in an ocular circulation is locally mediated, but the relative contributions of the underlying local control mechanisms are ill defined. Notwithstanding these caveats, there is evidence of local control in the prelaminar optic nerve, choroid retina, ciliary body and iris.

6.1 TYPES OF LOCAL CONTROL

Be definition, local control of blood flow refers to mechanisms intrinsic to the blood vessels and nearby parenchymal cells. These mechanisms include myogenic local control, metabolic local control, flow-mediated vasodilation and flow control by intercellular conduction.

6.2 MYOGENIC LOCAL CONTROL

"The muscular coat of the arteries reacts, like smooth muscle in other situations, to a stretching force by contraction. It also reacts to a diminution of tension by relaxation, shown, of course, only when in a state of tone. These reactions are independent of the central nervous system, and are of a myogenic nature." "The peripheral powers of reaction possessed by the arteries is of such a nature as to provide as far as possible for the maintenance of a constant flow of blood through the tissues supplied by them, whatever may be the height of the general blood-pressure, except in so far as they are directly overruled by impulses from the central nervous system." Baylis, 1902[29].

As Baylis observed over a century ago, vascular smooth muscle contracts in response to stretch and relaxes when imposed stretch is released, and this intrinsic behavior tends to promote constant blood flow despite changing arterial pressure. The myogenic mechanism, or myogenic response, occurs in vessels from diverse tissues and organs, including the eye (Fig 6.1). In vitro experiments indicate that the myogenic response requires extracellular calcium, but it does not require an intact endothelium (Fig 6.2). The myogenic response is also fast, occurring within seconds to minutes (Fig 6.3).

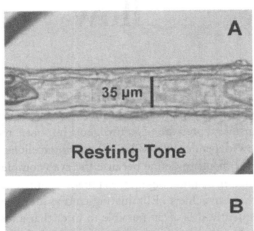

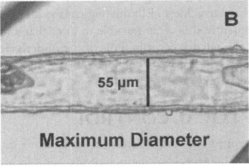

Figure 6.1: In vitro cannulated human retinal arteriole. (A) The vessel was allowed to develop resting basal tone (35 μm internal diameter) at 55 cm H2O intraluminal pressure. (B) Maximum diameter (55 μm internal diameter) of the vessel was established in calcium-free solution containing 0.1 mM sodium nitroprusside[30]. Reproduced with permission from Investigative Ophthalmology & Visual Sciences.

In many organs and tissues, blood flow is relatively stable over a range of arterial pressure in the absence of any neurohumoral input – a flow behavior known as autoregulation. As noted by Baylis, the myogenic mechanism has the potential to help maintain blood flow if arterial pressure changes, and there is considerable evidence supporting a myogenic role in autoregulation[35]. However, the myogenic mechanism responds to stretch, or more specifically vascular wall tension, and consequently, it can also exacerbate the flow response to a pressure change in some situations. For example, if venous pressure increases, the pressures upstream also increase and elicit an arterial myogenic response so that the fall in blood flow due to the decreased perfusion pressure is worsened by the myogenic

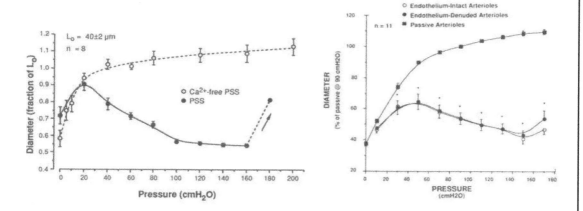

Figure 6.2: Vessel diameter responses to increasing intraluminal pressure. Left: hamster cheek pouch arterioles fail to constrict in response to increasing intraluminal pressure without extracellular calcium. Right: rat cremaster muscle arterioles constrict in response to increasing intraluminal pressure with and without endothelium[31,32]. Reproduced with permission from American Physiological Society.

vasoconstriction[36]. Figure 6.4 shows an example of myogenic non-autoregulatory behavior in a rat cremaster arteriole using the pressurized box preparation[37]. In this preparation, the animal is placed inside an airtight box and the cremaster muscle is exteriorized for viewing on an inverted microscope stage. When the box pressure is raised, there is an equal increase in arterial and venous pressures, so that the transmural pressure increases without altering the perfusion pressure gradient. This causes a robust myogenic response and fall in blood flow.

As Figure 6.4 demonstrates, the myogenic mechanism is dynamic, but it does not deliberately maintain constant blood flow. For the specific case of changing arterial pressure, Johnson proposed that myogenic autoregulation can occur when arterial smooth muscle incorporates a sensor responsive to changing wall tension coupled in series with the contractile elements and moderate feedback gain (Fig 6.5)[35,38]. This regulatory loop would permit the vessel radius adjustments necessary to maintain flow when pressure changes (e.g., if arterial pressure increases, the arterial contraction must decrease the radius below control to maintain blood flow constant). Johnson observed that in terms of homeostasis, the myogenic mechanism is better suited to regulating capillary hydrostatic pressure than blood flow (e.g., if arterial or venous pressure rise, the arterial myogenic vasoconstriction would act to preserve capillary hydrostatic pressure).

6.3   METABOLIC LOCAL CONTROL

The basic assumption of metabolic local control is that tissues regulate their blood flow to maintain nutrient delivery and waste removal consistent with metabolic demand (Fig 6.6)[39]. The underlying

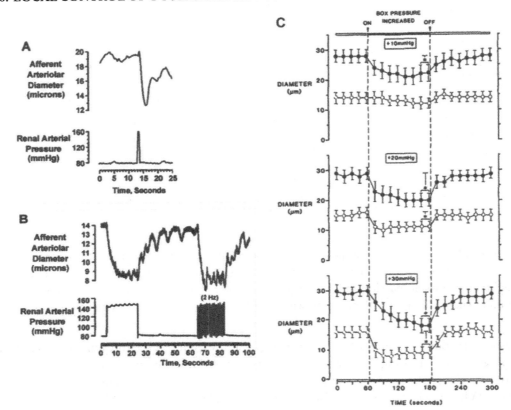

Figure 6.3: Speed of myogenic response. (A) Rapid afferent arteriole contractile responses of in vitro perfused hydronephrotic rat kidney preparation to a 1 sec arterial pressure spike and (B) to 20 sec sustained or pulsatile step-increases in arterial pressure. (C) In vivo rat cremaster 3rd order (filled circles) and 4th order (open circles) arteriole responses to step increases in transmural pressure of 10, 20 and 30 mmHg. Response rate and degree of constriction vary with location in vascular tree and size of pressure step[33,34]. Reproduced with permission from Circulation Research, Wolters Kluwer Health.

assumption is that communication occurs between parenchymal cells and the smooth muscle cells controlling the vascular resistance (arterioles) and capillary flow distribution (pre-capillary sphincters and pericytes)[40,41]. Because most tissues use aerobic metabolism, the oxygen delivery by blood flow to the tissue is often considered the regulated variable. If oxygen delivery decreases (e.g., due to a fall in arterial pressure) or oxygen demand increases (e.g., increased neuronal activity), the parenchymal cells produce a vasodilatory signal that increases tissue blood flow and capillary perfusion such that oxygen delivery is again matched to oxygen demand. Conversely, if oxygen delivery exceeds demand,

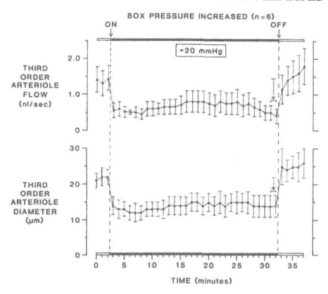

Figure 6.4: Myogenic response to increased transmural pressure at constant perfusion pressure in rat cremaster arteriole[34]. Reproduced with permission from Circulation Research, Wolters Kluwer Health.

the parenchymal cells decrease production of the vaosdilatory signal until delivery and demand are again matched. There are numerous vasodilator candidates linked to metabolism that can act as the feedback signal (e.g., adenosine, CO2, H+, lactate, etc.), and it is likely that all participate to a variable extent depending on the tissue.

Several pieces of evidence support the metabolic local control hypothesis: reactive hyperemia (Fig 6.7), functional hyperemia (Fig 6.8), modulation of pressure-flow autoregulation by metabolic stimulation (Fig 6.9), and hypoxic hyperemia (Fig 6.10).

6.4   FLOW-MEDIATED VASODILATION

In vitro and in vivo studies of large and small arteries indicate that increasing blood flow elicits an endothelium-dependent vasodilation (Fig 6.11)[46–50]. The data indicate that the response is mediated by shear stress exerted on the endothelial cells by the velocity and viscosity of blood moving within the vessel lumen (Fig 6.12). The response is inhibited by indomethacin (Fig 6.12) and nitric oxide synthase inhibitors, indicating that endothelial release of vasoactive prostaglandins and nitric oxide participate in the response[51,52]. The contribution of flow-mediated vasodilation in local control is complex since it has the potential to be inherently unstable (i.e., an increase in flow elicits a vasodilation that causes a further increase in flow). However, the response varies with location in the arterial tree and is likely counterbalanced by metabolic and myogenic local control.

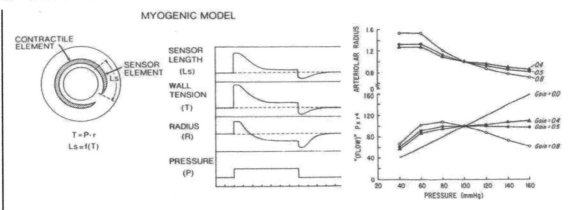

Figure 6.5: Model of myogenic autoregulation. Model assumes that resistance vessels have a sensor in series with the contractile element that responds to changes in wall tension as defined by the Law of LaPlace (tension equals the transmural pressure times the radius, T = Pr). The model addresses a theoretical issue for myogenic autoregulation, i.e., if the arterial wall is stretched by an increase in pressure, the muscle cannot simply contract back to its original length, since that would return the vessel to its original radius, resistance would be unchanged, and flow would increase. For flow to remain constant despite an increase in pressure, the muscle fibers need to shorten to less than their pre-stretched length, so that the radius is less than control and resistance increases. With moderate feedback gain, the model predicts autoregulatory flow behavior. However, if the gain is too high, the model predicts "super-regulation" where flow increases in response to decreased perfusion pressure[35,38]. Reproduced with permission from American Physiological Society.

6.5   FLOW CONTROL BY INTERCELLULAR CONDUCTION

One potential integrating mechanism for the various local control mechanisms is intercellular communication along the arterial tree[53]. The evidence for this mechanism is the rapid propagation of a focal vasodilation elicited by iontophoretic application of acetylcholine (Fig 6.13)[54]. The vasodilation spreads from one region of an artery or arteriole to another. The fact that the vasodilation spreads past an upstream occlusion indicates that flow-mediated vasodilation is not involved. The propagated vasodilation is associated with a hyperpolarization of the endothelial cells (Fig 6.14)[55].

6.6   OCULAR LOCAL CONTROL

The study of local control mechanisms in the ocular circulations is difficult because of the eye's unique anatomy and the limitations of current blood flow measuring technology. Nonetheless, there are clear examples of local control phenomena in each of the ocular circulations.

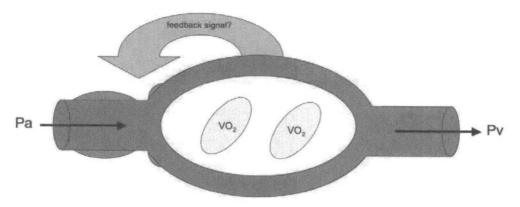

Figure 6.6: Model of metabolic local control. Arterial resistance and capillary perfusion are modulated by a feedback signal linked to parenchymal metabolism and oxygen consumption (VO2). (Pa: arterial pressure; Pv: venous pressure; arrows: direction of blood flow).

6.6.1   OPTIC NERVE HEAD (ONH)

Numerous studies provide evidence of autoregulation in the prelaminar ONH in different species with blood flow measured with different techniques and perfusion pressure varied by changing IOP or blood pressure (Fig 6.15)[56–59]. However, the underlying mechanisms responsible for this behavior are unclear, though metabolic and myogenic mechanisms seem most likely.

Several pieces of evidence indicate metabolic control in ONH autoregulation. First, the ONH has a strong functional hyperemic response during retinal illumination with a flickering light stimulus (Fig 6.16)[60]. The functional hyperemia is linked to metabolism since it is associated with a decrease in ONH PO2 indicative of increased oxygen consumption and increased interstitial potassium concentration consistent with increased nerve activity[61]. Local NO production also increases and may contribute, although the functional hyperemia persists despite nitric oxide synthase inhibition[62]. The response is also altered by exogenous adenosine, but it is unclear whether endogenous adenosine is involved[62]. Second, the pressure-flow relationship is shifted upwards during metabolic stimulation (Fig 6.17)[63]. Interestingly, the break-point in the pressure-flow relationship occurs at a higher perfusion pressure than in control. This may be due to fewer action potentials arriving from the retina due to insufficient retinal perfusion or the vasodilatory reserve may be exhausted sooner at the higher metabolic rate (i.e., the ONH arterioles have a maximum achievable diameter all of which is available to respond to decreased perfusion pressure under control conditions, but less is available when doubly challenged by increased metabolism and decreased perfusion pressure). Third, ONH blood flow decreases during hyperoxia and increases during hypoxia (Fig 6.18)[64]. Lastly, the ONH appears to undergo a reactive hyperemia following brief periods of ischemia, at least in some species (Fig 6.19)[63]. Reactive hyperemia seems to occur in cats, monkeys and humans[65], but the

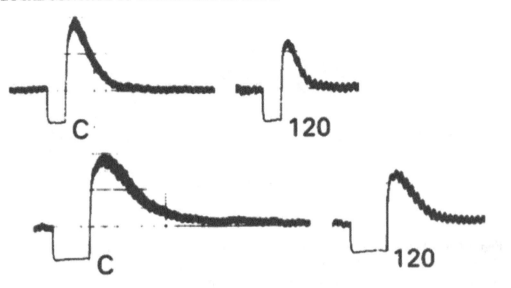

Figure 6.7: Reactive hyperemia. Blood flow response in canine circumflex artery upon release of 15 sec (top) and 30 sec (bottom) arterial occlusions before (left) and after (right) giving a non-selective adenosine antagonist (theophylline). Extent of post-occlusion blood flow overshoot increases with occlusion duration and is decreased by adenosine antagonist [42]. Reproduced with permission from British Journal of Parmacology, Wiley.

experiments were not designed specifically to study reactive hyperemia (i.e., the ischemia duration was not varied systematically or done at different levels of metabolic activity). Taken together, these lines of evidence support the involvement of metabolic local control in the ONH.

There is also evidence against metabolic involvement in ONH local control, at least in the rabbit (Fig 6.20). In that species, a 10 min period of relative ischemia did not elicit a reactive hyperemic response, although there was clear evidence of autoregulation (i.e., the relative decrease in ONH velocity was much smaller than the relative decrease in perfusion pressure) [68]. Moreover, the speed of the autoregulatory response in the rabbit to a step-decrease in perfusion pressure was quite rapid (<5 sec), which seems fast for the accumulation of vasoactive metabolites and perhaps more in keeping with a myogenic response (though the flicker response, which is clearly metabolic, is also quite fast) [69]. The difference in the reactive hyperemic responses in the rabbit versus the cat and monkey may reflect species differences, but more studies designed specifically to identify the local control mechanisms responsible for ONH autoregulation are clearly needed.

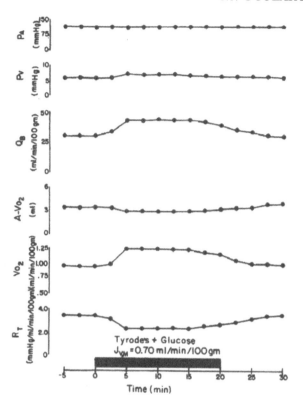

Figure 6.8: Functional hyperemia. Blood flow (Qb) response in an isolated segment of feline ileum before, during and after filling the lumen with a glucose solution. Oxygen consumption (VO2) increased during glucose absorption. The increased VO2 was achieved by increased Qb rather than increased arteriovenous oxygen extraction (A-V O2). The increased Qb was mediated by a decrease in vascular resistance (Rt) since arterial (Pa) and venous (Pv) pressures were unaffected[43]. Reproduced with permission from American Physiological Society.

6.6.2   CHOROID

The evidence regarding choroidal autoregulation has varied over the years. The advent of the microsphere technique for use in the eye[70] in the early 1970's stimulated studies of choroidal responses to changing perfusion pressure, typically by raising IOP. In some cases, the results indicated no choroidal autoregulation, as in a cat study by Alm and Bill, while another cat study by Weiter et al. showed the choroid has autoregulatory ability (Fig 6.21)[71,72]. In another study by Alm and Bill, the results in primates were ambiguous (Fig 6.22)[73].

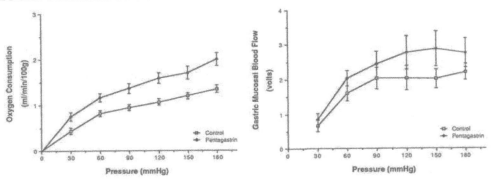

Figure 6.9: Metabolic activity and autoregulation. Effect perfusion pressure on oxygen consumption and mucosal blood flow in an isolated canine stomach preparation before and during pentagastrin-stimulated acid secretion. Increased oxygen consumption paralleled by an upward shift in the mucosal pressure-flow relationship[44]. Reproduced with permission from Gastroenterology, Elsevier.

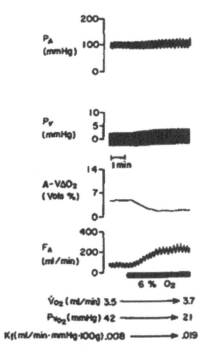

Figure 6.10: Hypoxic vasodilation. Effect of systemic hypoxia on canine skeletal muscle blood flow in an areflexic dog preparation[45]. Reproduced with permission from Circulation Research, Wolters Kluwer Health.

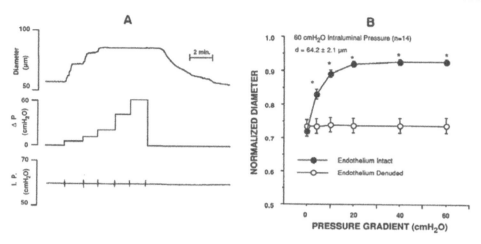

Figure 6.11: Flow-mediated vasodilation. In vitro porcine coronary arterioles dilate in response to flow achieved by step-increases in perfusion pressure (ΔP) without changing the mid-point intraluminal pressure (A). Flow-induced dilation is endothelium-dependent (B)[50]. Reproduced with permission from American Physiological Society.

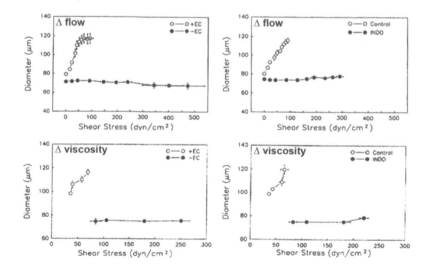

Figure 6.12: Shear stress and flow-mediated vasodilation. In vitro rat cremaster arterioles dilate in response to shear stress increased by raising flow (top) or viscosity (bottom). Shear stress response is abolished by endothelial removal (left) or indomethacin (right)[51]. Reproduced with permission from Circulation Research, Wolters Kluwer Health.

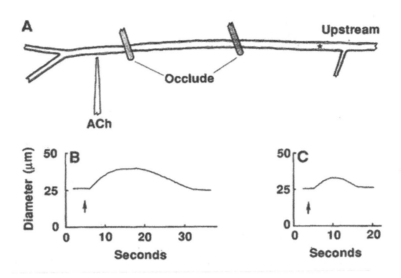

Figure 6.13: Propagated vasodilation. In hamster cheek pouch arterioles, a focal acetylcholine induced vasodilation propagates upstream past a double occlusion indicating intercellular communication along the arterial tree[54].

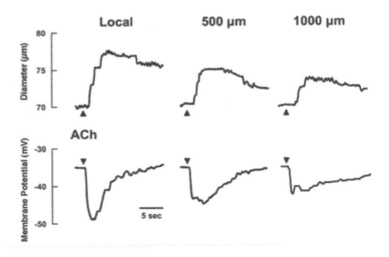

Figure 6.14: Propagated vasodilation associated with hyperpolarization of endothelial membrane potential[55]. Reproduced with permission from American Physiological Society.

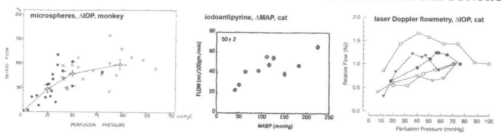

Figure 6.15: Optic nerve head autoregulation observed in different species with different blood flow measuring technique and difference perfusion pressure perturbations [56–58]. Reproduced with permission from Investigative Ophthalmology & Visual Science.

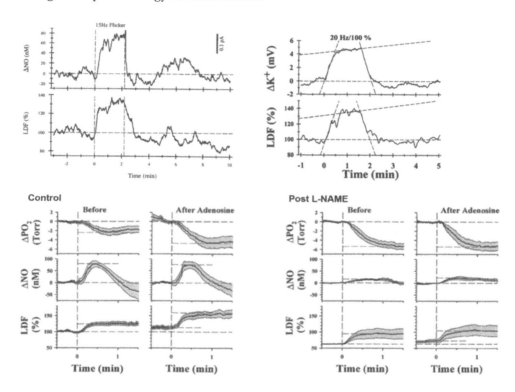

Figure 6.16: ONH functional hyperemia. (Top, left) Flickering light stimulation of the retina in the anesthetized cat elicits an increase in ONH nitric oxide (NO) and ONH blood flow measured by LDF. (Top, right) Retinal flicker in the cat also increases ONH potassium levels and ONH blood flow. (Bottom) Cat retinal flicker responses are modulated by exogenous adenosine and nitric oxide synthase inhibition with L-NAME [61,62,66]. Reproduced with permission from Investigative Ophthalmology & Visual Science.

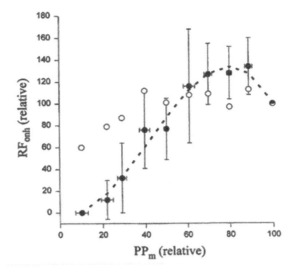

Figure 6.17: Metabolic stimulation and ONH autoregulation. The cat ONH pressure-flow relationship obtained by raising IOP during flicker (closed circles) and without (open circles) flicker. (RFonh: ONH blood flow response measured by LDF)[63]. Reproduced with permission from Microvascular Research, Elsevier.

Because they used femoral arterial pressure as an index of ophthalmic artery pressure, the authors noted "If the line connecting the values for the two eyes is extrapolated and then intercepts either the positive flow axis or the positive pressure axis below 25 cm H_2O [18.4 mmHg] this suggests a vasodilation in the eye with reduced perfusion pressure.... Although some lines point towards the positive flow axis the mean result does not indicate any marked reduction in vascular resistance in response to a reduction in perfusion pressure." Using the authors' definition, roughly half the animals autoregulated and the other half did not (Fig 6.22). Given the lack of clear evidence of autoregulation, the authors concluded that the choroid was passive. Other studies came to a similar conclusion.

Clearer evidence of autoregulation in the choroid came later from rabbit studies using a fiber optic-based laser Doppler flowmeter (Fig 6.23)[17,74,75]. In those studies, the efficacy of choroidal autoregulation depended on the method used to vary the perfusion pressure, i.e., autoregulation occurred over a wider perfusion pressure range when arterial pressure was manipulated without controlling IOP than when MAP was raised at a constant IOP or IOP was raised at a constant MAP. It was also noted that the efficacy of choroidal autoregulation depended on the method of anesthesia, i.e., autoregulation occurred under pentobarbital anesthesia but was largely abolished by

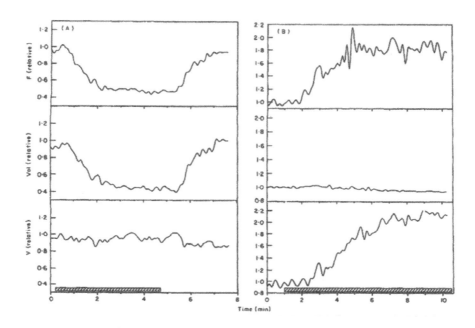

Figure 6.18: Cat ONH responses to hyperoxia (left) and hypoxia (right) measured by LDF[67] (F: blood flow: Vol: index of number of moving blood cells; V: mean velocity of moving blood cells). Reproduced with permission from Experimental Eye Research, Elsevier.

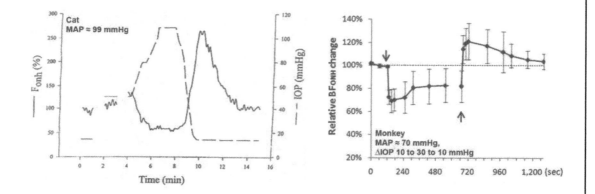

Figure 6.19: Reactive hyperemia measured by LDF in the optic nerve head of cat (left) and monkey (right)[59,63]. Reproduced with permission from Microvascular Research, Elsevier.

Nembutal, which contains 40% propylene glycol and 10% alcohol[76]. Methodological issues such as these and others may account for the discrepant evidence for choroidal autoregulation.

In contrast to the optic nerve and retina, the choroid is richly innervated, and so an interaction of local and neural control mechanisms is inherent in the choroidal response to changing perfusion pressure. Consequently, designating a choroidal blood flow response to changing perfusion pressure as autoregulation (i.e., due solely to local control) may not be appropriate. For that reason, some authors prefer the term "baroregulation" when all regulatory mechanisms are intact and choroidal blood flow does not change with perfusion pressure. However, in animals it is possible to minimize the neural control contribution by systemic ganglionic blockade (Fig 6.24). In rabbits, this causes a slight downward shift in the choroidal pressure-flow relationship, but choroidal blood flow still remains pressure-independent until perfusion pressure falls below approximately 40 mmHg[75]. This result indicates that the choroid is capable of autoregulation. However, the downward shift in the pressure-flow relation with ganglionic blockade also indicates a degree of tonic neural vasodilator tone. Some of that tone may be nitridergic, since inhibition of nitric oxide synthase (NOS) with L-NAME also causes a downward shift in the pressure-flow relationship (Fig 6.24); however, L-NAME is a non-selective NOS inhibitor and much of the downward shift is likely due to the loss of endothelial NOS vasodilatory tone. The underlying vasoconstrictor tone revealed by NOS inhibition

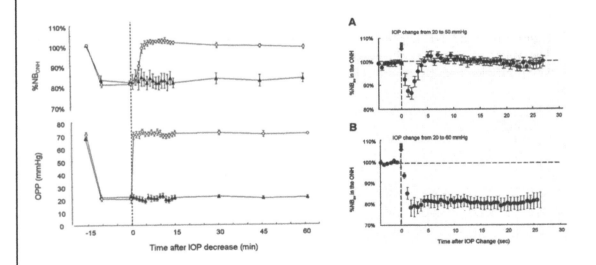

Figure 6.20: Evidence against ONH metabolic local control. (Left) Rabbit ONH blood velocity (by laser speckle flowgraphy) response to decreasing ocular perfusion pressure (OPP) by raising IOP shows autoregulation but no reactive hyperemia upon restoration of OPP to control. (Right) Rabbit ONH autoregulatory response to increasing IOP occurs within 5 sec.[68,69]. Reproduced with permission from Investigative Ophthalmology & Visual Science.

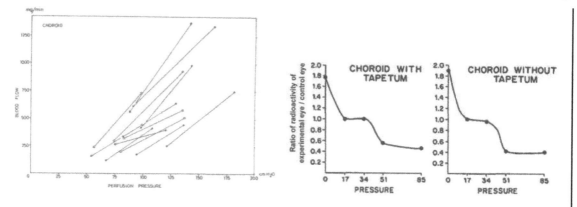

Figure 6.21: Early evidence against (left) and for (right) choroidal autoregulation based on binocular microsphere measurements in cats with IOP elevated in one eye. (Perfusion Pressure = MAP − IOP; Pressure = IOP)[71,72]. Reproduced with permission from Acta Phisiology, Wiley Blackwell.

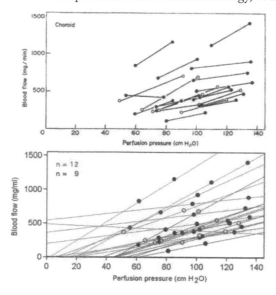

Figure 6.22: Ambiguous evidence for and against choroidal autoregulation based on binocular microsphere measurements in primates with IOP elevated in one eye. Lines connect the data points for the eyes of each monkey. Threshold for autoregulation occurs at perfusion pressure of 25 cm H2O, with lines intersecting the x-axis below that threshold indicating autoregulation. (Top: original figure; Bottom: redrawn figure with linear regression lines)[73]. Reproduced with permission from Experimental Eye Research, Elsevier.

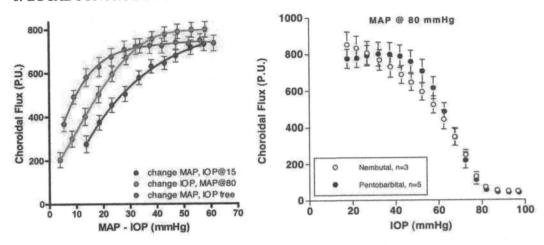

Figure 6.23: Efficacy of choroidal autoregulation in the rabbit depends on method used to manipulate perfusion pressure (left) and method of anesthesia (right)[17,76]. Reproduced with permission from Investigative Ophthalmology & Visual Science.

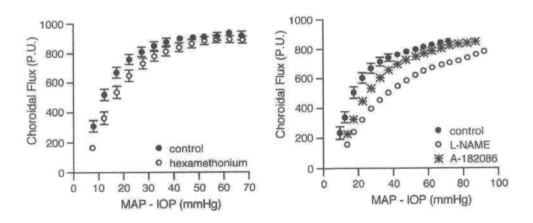

Figure 6.24: Inhibition of neural control by ganglionic blockade with hexamethonium causes a modest downward shift in the pressure-flow relationship but flow remains pressure-independent over a wide pressure range, indicating the autoregulatory behavior is locally mediated. Non-selective NOS inhibition with L-NAME elicits a marked downward shift in the pressure-flow relationship that is largely reversed by non-selective endothelin antagonism indicating significant roles of nitric oxide and endothelin in choroidal blood flow regulation[75]. Reproduced with permission from Experimental Eye Research, Elsevier.

seems to be due to endothelin, since the L-NAME induced downward shift is largely reversed by the non-selective endothelin antagonist, A-182086[75,77].

Metabolic local control does not seem to play a role in choroidal autoregulation since the choroid does not respond markedly to retinal metabolic stimulation by flicker or to hyperoxia, though it does respond to hypocapnia (Fig 6.25)[78,79]. Other studies report a hyperemic response to hypercapnia[71,80]. The choroid also does not exhibit a reactive hyperemic response to brief (Fig 6.26) or long periods of ischemia[81]. Choroidal blood flow also does not increase (and may even decrease) when retinal oxygen consumption increases in the dark such that the inner photoreceptor layer becomes nearly anoxic (see below). The apparent absence of choroidal metabolic local control may be due to the high flow rate in the choroid and its anatomical organization. Metabolic local control is thought to depend on metabolic vasodilators reaching the resistance vessels. The choroid itself has little parenchymal metabolism, so the source of metabolic vasodilators would be the RPE and photoreceptors. The sheet-like choriocapillaris design is thought to optimize oxygen delivery and waste removal for the RPE and photoreceptors. If efficient, the waste removal function of the choriocapillaris would preclude vasodilators from the RPE and photoreceptors from reaching the choroidal arterioles. This is one plausible explanation for the lack of choroidal metabolic local control.

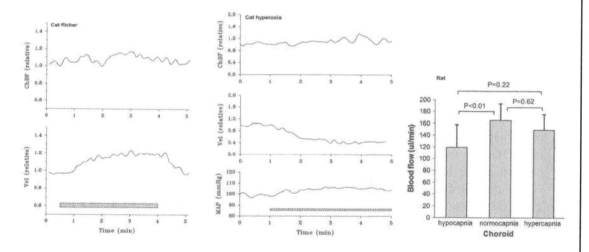

Figure 6.25: Minimal choroidal blood flow responses to retinal flickering light stimulation (left), hyperoxia (middle) or hypercapnia (right) indicate little metabolic local control[78,79]. Reproduced with permission from Experimental Eye Research, Elsevier.

There is some evidence for choroidal myogenic local control, at least in the rabbit[24,74]. To explore whether a myogenic mechanism could account for choroidal autoregulatory-like behavior in the rabbit, Kiel and Shepherd[74] created a mathematical model incorporating myogenic control of choroidal arterial resistance and passive (Starling resistor) control of choroidal venous resistance.

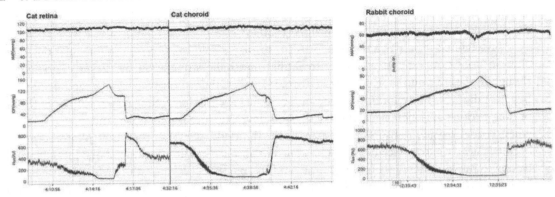

Figure 6.26: Lack of choroidal reactive hyperemia indicates little metabolic local control. (Author's unpublished observations. MAP: mean arterial pressure; IOP: intraocular pressure; Flux: blood flow by LDF).

The model simulated pressure-flow relationship was similar to that found in vivo, suggesting that a myogenic mechanism could account for the autoregulatory-like behavior. Moreover, the model predicted decreased choroidal blood flow in response to increased perfusion pressure in conditions conducive to heightened wall tension, and similar responses were found in vivo (Fig 6.27). Thus, it appears myogenic local control may be operative in the choroid.

As noted earlier, from a functional perspective, the myogenic mechanism is better suited to regulating capillary hydrostatic pressure than blood flow. If so, a myogenic mechanism in the choroid could help to stabilize blood volume during arterial pressure fluctuations and so minimize fluctuations in IOP. Consistent with this idea, the IOP normally rises a few mmHg in response to a 30-40 mmHg mechanically induced increase in arterial pressure, but if vascular control is blocked with a systemic vasodilator, the IOP response to a similar arterial pressure increase is much greater (Fig 6.28)[24]. This IOP protective response occurs during autonomic blockade, so it has a local mechanism. If the arterial hypertension is neurally or humorally mediated, the local mechanism may augment the choroidal vasoconstriction relative to that occurring throughout the systemic circulation[82].

A function proposed for the choroidal circulation that may have a local component is retinal temperature regulation. Given the small amount of metabolically active tissue (i.e., heat generating) relative to the size of the globe, the temperatures of the retina and the eye are primarily determined by the blood-borne convective heat delivery from the core and heat dissipation from the exposed ocular surface. As the largest of the ocular circulations, the choroid provides most of the convective heat delivery to the eye. In an environment cooler than core body temperature, the thermal gradient favors ocular heat loss; conversely, in a hot environment, the thermal gradient favors ocular heat gain. An additional source of heat gain is light absorption in the pigmented RPE and choroid. Given these thermodynamic parameters, it follows that eye temperature will fall if ocular blood flow is

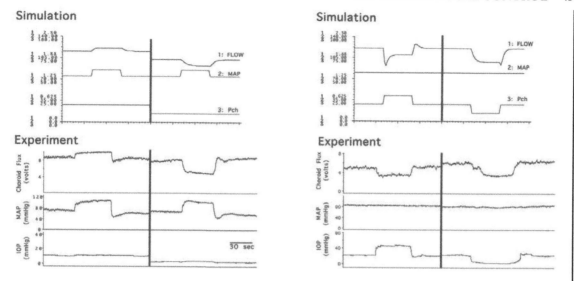

Figure 6.27: Model simulations and confirmatory evidence of choroidal myogenic local control[74]. Reproduced with permission from Investigative Ophthalmology & Visual Science.

reduced in a cold environment, or rise if the environment is hot. If the temperature outside the eye is the same as core body temperature, stopping ocular blood flow will not change retinal temperature.

Parver et al. reported results from two monkeys in which raising IOP above systolic blood pressure decreased the temperature of a thermistor inside a 23 gauge needle inserted in the retina-choroid by 1° - 1.2° C[83]. The temperatures of the environment, the saline drip on the cornea, and the infusate used to raise IOP were not provided so the thermal gradients are unclear. Given that the retina-choroid temperatures were measured at the macula where the thermal gradient should be dominated by the temperature of the orbit, the magnitude and speed (i.e., "not less than one minute after alteration of the pressure") of the retina-choroid temperature decreases suggest that the thermal gradient to the exposed anterior eye surface must have been quite large. In the same two monkeys, exposure of the cornea to 1.09 mW/cm^2 of light caused an increase in retina-choroid temperature of ≈ 0.9°C when the IOP was set at 20 mmHg, which increased another ≈ 0.8°C when IOP was raised above systolic blood pressure.

Based on these results, the authors suggested "that the high flow choroidal circulation normally functions to stabilize the temperature environment of the retinal pigment epithelium and outer retinal layers."[83] A problem with this suggestion is that the temperature of choroidal blood is set by the core body temperature, which can vary significantly. For example, walking for 30 min in a cool environment followed by walking for 1 hr in a hot environment can raise core body temperature by 3.5°C (Fig 6.29)[84]. Thus, in addition to the thermal gradient mentioned earlier, the ability of the

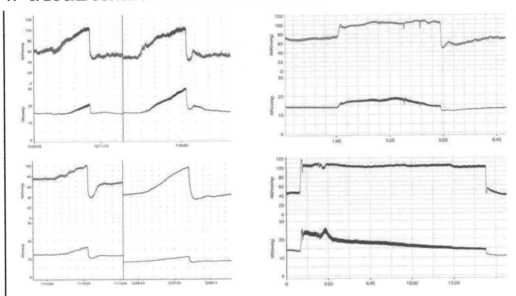

Figure 6.28: Protection of the eye from arterial pressure-dependent changes in IOP is a possible function of choroidal myogenic local control. (Left, top) IOP responses to acute ramp increase in MAP before and after systemic vasodilation with hydralazine. (Left, bottom) IOP responses to acute ramp increase in MAP before and after ganglionic blockade with hydralazine. (Right) IOP responses to sustained MAP increase under control conditions (top) and after systemic vasodilation (bottom). All traces obtained in anesthetized rabbits with MAP controlled mechanically with hydraulic aortic occluders. (MAP: mean arterial pressure; IOP: intraocular pressure)[24]. Reproduced with permission from Experimental Eye Research, Elsevier.

choroid to stabilize retinal temperature depends greatly on whole body thermoregulation. Moreover, the 0.9°C increase in retina-choroid temperature upon light exposure with IOP at 20 mmHg, suggests that choroidal blood flow does a poor job of stabilizing retinal temperature. Indeed, some of that increase in temperature may have been a light-induced reflex since Parver et al. found that light applied to the contralateral eye increased ipsilateral retina-choroid and scleral temperature as well as an index of choroidal blood flow; the reflex, presumably, also works when the ipsilateral eye is light exposed[85]. Such a reflex suggests that choroidal blood flow is not regulated to maintain retinal temperature.

6.6.3 RETINA

Evidence for autoregulation of retinal blood flow is found in various species with different blood flow measuring techniques and methods of perfusion pressure manipulation (Fig 6.30). Given its

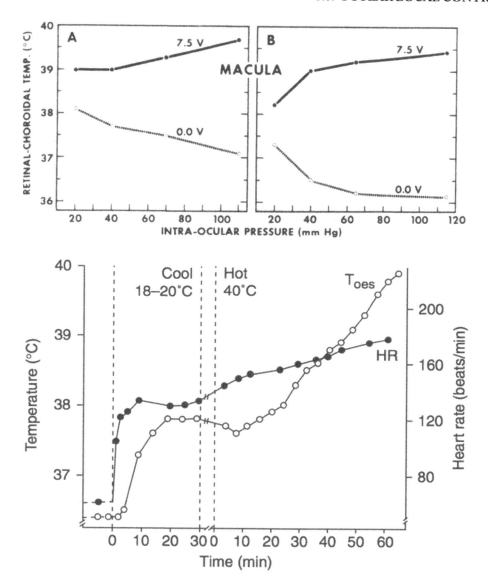

Figure 6.29: Choroidal blood flow and retinal temperature. (Top) effect of light (lamp powered with 7.5V) and darkness (0.0 V) on retinal temperature as choroidal blood flow is reduced by raising IOP in two monkey eyes. (Bottom) changes in core body temperature (T_{oes}) and heart rate (HR) during walking in a cool and hot environment. Reproduced with permission from American Journal of Ophthalmology, Elsevier.

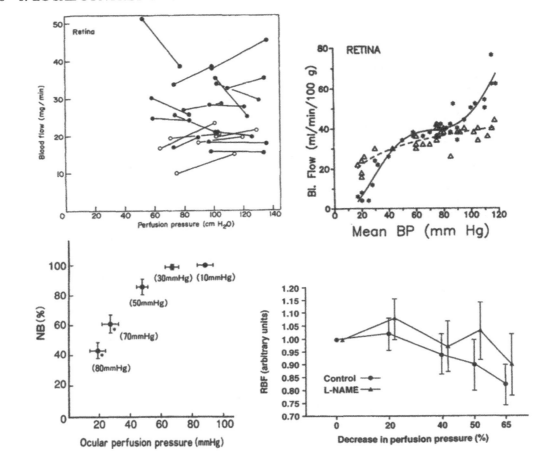

Figure 6.30: Autoregulation of retinal blood flow in monkey (top left), piglet before (circles) and after (triangles) ibuprofen (top right), rabbit (bottom left) and cat before and after L-NAME[71,73,86–88]. Reproduced with permission from Acta Phisiology, Wiley Blackwell.

lack of autonomic innervation and high metabolic needs, autoregulation of retinal blood flow is not surprising. However, local control in the retina is complex. In many species, retinal nutrient delivery and waste removal are provided by both retinal and choroidal circulations, but some species subsist with a negligible retinal circulation (e.g., rabbits), others have none (e.g., guinea pigs), and the primate foveal region is devoid of retinal vessels despite its high density of metabolically active photoreceptors. Obviously, the link between retinal perfusion and metabolism is complicated, and varies by species and location, which makes understanding metabolic local control difficult. The negative visual consequences of retinal edema underscore the likely importance of myogenic local

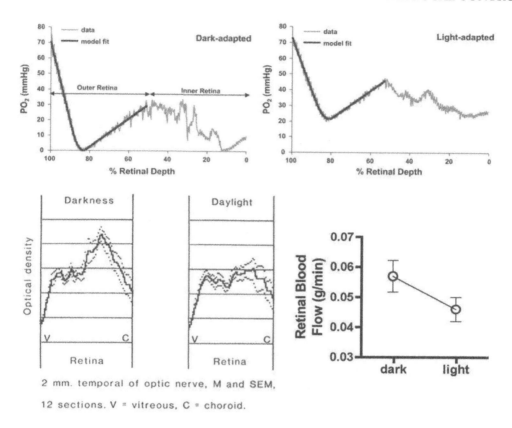

Figure 6.31: Effect of light on retinal metabolism and blood flow[93] (data for lower right graph from Table 1[93]). Reproduced with permission from Eye, Nature.

control, but this mechanism is difficult to study in the in vivo retina though it is evident under in vitro conditions (Fig 6.1). The contributions of flow mediated vasodilation and intercellular conduction are even harder to study and less well understood. Thus, while the evidence for retinal metabolic local control predominates, the other forms of local control may contribute as well.

A counterintuitive phenomenon in the retina is that oxygen consumption rises in the dark due to increased Na/K ATPase activity[89,90]. In species with a dual retinal blood supply (i.e., retinal and choroidal circulations), the dark stimulated increase in oxygen consumption is sufficient to lower the PO2 of the photoreceptor inner segments to near zero (Fig 6.31)[91,92]. There is a corresponding increase in glucose consumption in approximately the same location in the dark, and retinal blood

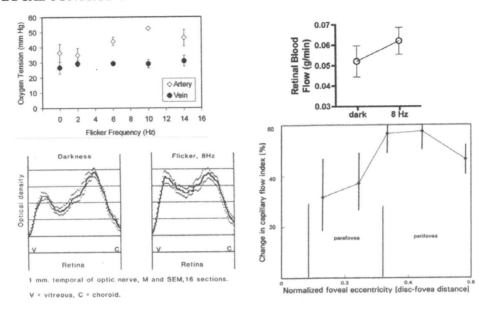

Figure 6.32: Retinal stimulation with flickering light increases retinal metabolism, as indicated by increased aterio-venous oxygen difference (top left) and increased inner retinal glucose uptake (bottom left), which elicits a retinal functional hyperemia (right top and bottom)[93–95] (data for upper right graph from Table 1[93]). Reproduced with permission from Eye, Nature.

flow is also higher in the dark[93]. This behavior appears to be an example of functional hyperemia, even though the metabolic activation occurs in the outer retina while the blood flow response occurs in the inner retina.

A clearer example of functional hyperemia is the retinal response to flickering light stimulation (Fig 6.32). In this case, the increase in retinal blood flow is associated with increased oxygen consumption indicated by the arteriovenous oxygen difference in paired retinal arteries and veins as well as increased glucose consumption in the inner retina[93–95]. Interestingly, there appears to be the greatest increase in retinal blood flow in the area with the highest density of ganglion cells, consistent with a link between metabolic demand and perfusion[95]. Additional evidence indicating significant retinal metabolic local control include the increase in retinal blood flow in response to hypoxia[96] and hypercapnia[97] as well as the decrease in blood flow in response to hyperoxia[98,99] (Fig 6.33) and the reactive hyperemia after brief (Fig 6.26) and long periods of ischemia (Fig 6.34)[81]. Surprisingly, the retinal pressure-flow relationships under light and dark-adapted conditions have not been determined, but it seems likely that the dark-adapted curve would be shifted upwards due to the

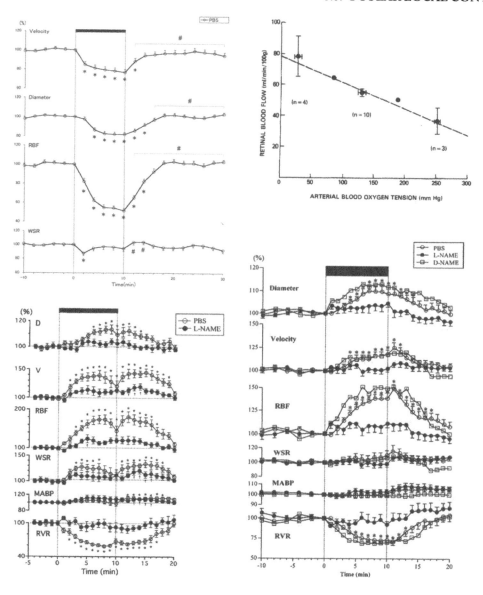

Figure 6.33: Retinal blood flow responses in cats consistent with metabolic local control. Retinal blood flow decreases in response to hyperoxia (top left and right) and increases in response to hypoxia (bottom left) and hypercapnia (bottom right)[96–99]. Reproduced with permission from Experimental Eye Research, Elsevier.

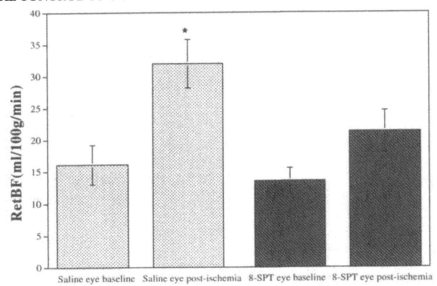

Figure 6.34: Retinal reactive hyperemia response after 1 hr of ischemia attenuated by adenosine receptor blockade with 8-sulfophenyltheophylline (8-SPT)[81]. Reproduced with permission from Current Eye Research, Taylor and Francis.

heightened oxygen consumption. Similarly, reactive hyperemic responses to brief ischemic periods would be expected to be larger in the dark.

6.6.4   CILIARY BODY

While the retina has basically one function (converting light information for the central nervous system) and a dual blood supply, the ciliary body has two functions (accommodation and aqueous secretion) with a single blood supply. Differentiating ciliary muscle and secretory tissue is fairly simple by histology, but complicated in vivo, and measuring the blood flow to the two tissue types is even harder. Microsphere measurements at normal and elevated IOP indicate that ciliary muscle and ciliary processes both autoregulate, but the flow readings vary significantly, possibly because of the small number of spheres that can be trapped in such a small amount of tissue (Fig 6.35).

LDF measurements in the rabbit also provide evidence of ciliary autoregulation, although it is also clear that the ciliary circulation is under neural control, since ganglionic blockade caused an upward and leftward shift in the pressure-flow relationship indicating tonic neuroconstrictor tone (Fig 6.36). This is an interesting example of the interplay between neural and local control. Ciliary blood flow provides the oxygen and nutrient delivery to support aqueous production, and ciliary blood flow can decrease approximately 30% before aqueous production is compromised under control

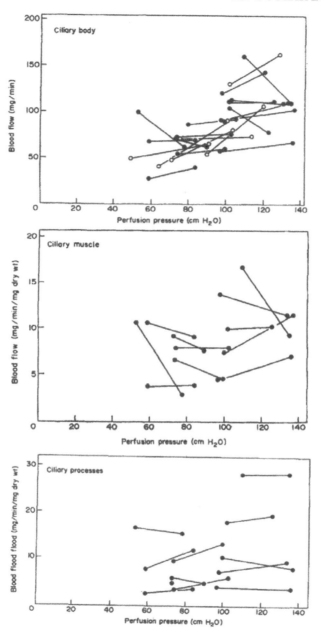

Figure 6.35: Evidence of autoregulation of ciliary blood flow in the cat[73]. Reproduced with permission from Experimental Eye Research, Elsevier.

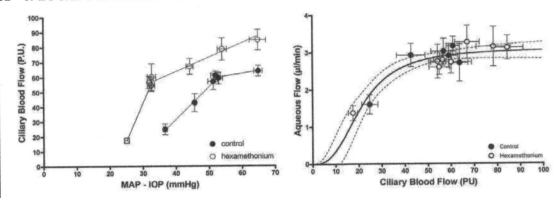

Figure 6.36: Rabbit ciliary pressure-flow relationship is shifted up and to the left by ganglionic blockade with hexamethonium, but the relationship between ciliary blood flow and aqueous flow is unaffected[100]. Reproduced with permission from Progress in Retinal and Eye Research, Elsevier.

conditions. It may be this perfusion reserve that makes possible the constrained autoregulatory range seen when both neural and local control are operative. The local mechanisms involved in ciliary autoregulation have not been investigated systematically, but the author has rarely seen flow behavior suggestive of metabolic local control. For example, ciliary blood flow does not undergo a reactive hyperemic response following periods of ischemia (Fig 6.37).

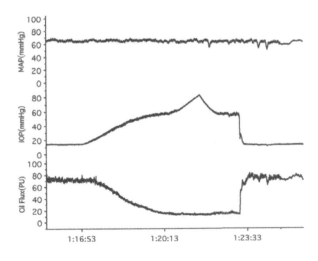

Figure 6.37: Absence of ciliary reactive hyperemia after ischemia in rabbit suggest little metabolic local control (author's unpublished observation).

6.6.5   IRIS

There are only a few published studies of iris blood flow in animals or humans. Microsphere measurements in primates indicate the iris autoregulates, but the measurements were quite variable (Fig 6.38). Laser speckle flowgraphy measurements in pigmented rabbits suggest little iris autoregulatory ability (Fig 6.38). Human iris blood flow also does not appear to autoregulate, but oddly there is evidence of iridial reactive hyperemia[101]. Given the limited number of studies, definitive comments on iris local control require addition data.

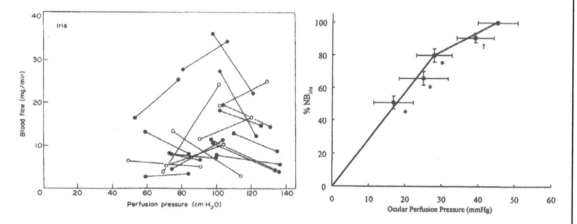

Figure 6.38: Iris blood flow responses to decreasing perfusion pressure by raising IOP in the monkey (left) and rabbit (right)[73,102]. Reproduced with permission from Experimental Eye Research, Elsevier.

Defining local control behavior and identifying the underlying mechanisms and their interactions is challenging even in more accessible vascular beds, but it is particularly hard in the ocular circulations. Local control clearly occurs in the eye, and further study will broaden our knowledge of its role in normal ocular function and disease.

CHAPTER 7

Neural control of ocular blood flow

As noted earlier, autonomic innervation is restricted to the vessels of the uvea (i.e., the choroid, ciliary body and iris) and optic nerve, while the retina appears to lack autonomic input. As in most tissues, the sympathetic nerves mediate uveal vasoconstriction (Fig 7.1); however, there is evidence that a non-adrenergic co-transmitter (possibly neuropeptide y) is also involved since phenoxybenzamine fails to abolish the response to sympathetic stimulation (Fig 7.2)[103].

Unlike most tissues, the parasympathetic nerves also play a role in controlling uveal blood flow. As might be expected, parasympathetic stimulation elicits vasodilation, though it seems more than just acetylcholine is involved as the neurotransmitter since the cholinergic antagonist atropine fails to abolish the response. Likely candidates include nitric oxide and vasoactive intestinal peptide (VIP).

Although the neural pathways and some of the neurotransmitters regulating uveal blood flow have been identified, what remains perplexing is their function. The uveal sympathetic nerves do not seem to participate in the arterial baroreflex; instead, they may play a protective role by preventing uveal over-perfusion during episodes of arterial hypertension brought on by generalized sympathetic activation[82]. The uveal parasympathetic nerves appear to modulate uveal blood flow during changing lighting conditions, but the ocular benefits of this response are unclear and require further study.

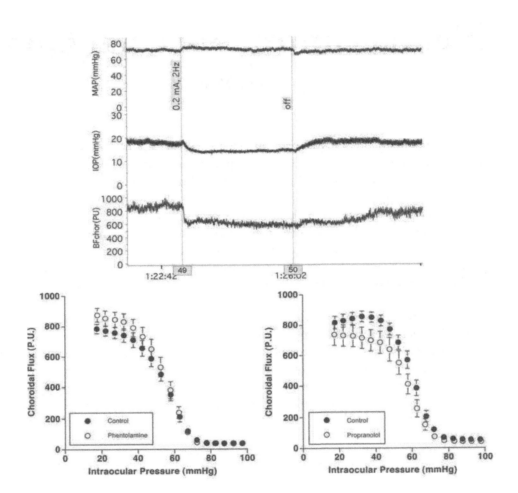

Figure 7.1: Sympathetic control of choroidal blood flow. (Top) direct electrical stimulation of rabbit cervical sympathetic nerve elicits a prompt vasoconstriction and decrease in choroidal blood flow. (Bottom) There appears to be tonic sympathetic tone in the rabbit since alpha-adrenergic blockade with phentolamine shifts the pressure-flow relationship upwards and beta-adrenergic blockade with propranolol shifts the relationship downwards[76]. Reproduced with permission from Investigative Ophthalmology & Visual Science.

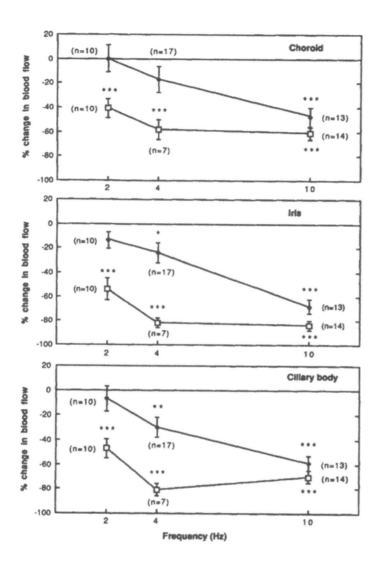

Figure 7.2: Sympathetic stimulation at different frequencies decreases blood flow in the rabbit choroid, iris and ciliary body, which is only partially blocked by alpha adrenergic blockade. (open squares: control; closed diamonds: post-phenoxybenzamine)[103]. Reproduced with permission from European Journal of Pharmacology, Elsevier.

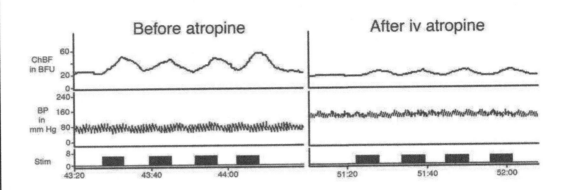

Figure 7.3: Electric stimulation of Edinger-Westphal nucleus elicits an increase in pigeon choroidal blood flow that is largely abolished by cholinergic blockade with intravenous atropine[104]. Reproduced with permission from Experimental Eye Research, Elsevier.

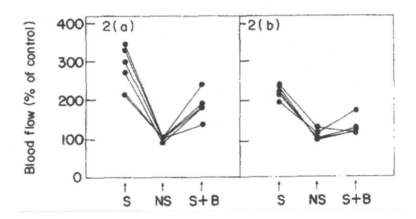

Figure 7.4: Electrical stimulation of facial nerve elicits an increase in cat choroidal blood flow that is partially blocked by atropine (left) and almost completely blocked by ganglionic blockade with hexamethonium[105]. Reproduced with permission from Experimental Eye Research, Elsevier.

CHAPTER 8

Summary

The ocular circulation is uniquely adapted for the eye's visual function. The need for a surrogate circulation of aqueous humor to nourish avascular tissues combined with the need to keep the eye inflated are challenges elegantly solved by the generation of the intraocular pressure, but at the cost of a much reduced perfusion pressure available to drive blood through the vessels of the eye. Much is known about how the ocular circulation is controlled and how it responds to its ever-changing conditions, and yet much more remains to be discovered to bring an end to blinding eye diseases such as glaucoma, age-related macular degeneration, diabetic retinopathy, retinopathy of prematurity and others that affect the ocular circulation.

Bibliography

[1] Reitsamer H A, Kiel J W. Effects of dopamine on ciliary blood flow, aqueous production, and intraocular pressure in rabbits. *Invest Ophthalmol Vis Sci.* 2002; 43: 2697 - 2703. 6

[2] Yu D. Y., Cringle S. J. Low oxygen consumption in the inner retina of the visual streak of the rabbit *Am J Physiol Heart Circ Physiol.* 2004; 286: H419–23. DOI: 10.1152/ajpheart.00643.2003 6, 43

[3] Kawaguchi I., Higashide T., Ohkubo S., Takeda H., Sugiyama K. In vivo imaging and quantitative evaluation of the rat retinal nerve fiber layer using scanning laser ophthalmoscopy *Invest Ophthalmol Vis Sci.* 2006; 47: 2911–6. DOI: 10.1167/iovs.05-1169 6

[4] Snodderly D. M., Weinhaus R. S., Choi J. C. Neural-vascular relationships in central retina of macaque monkeys (Macaca fascicularis) *J Neurosci.* 1992; 12: 1169–93. 7

[5] Risco J. M., Nopanitaya W. Ocular microcirculation. Scanning electron microscopic study *Invest Ophthalmol Vis Sci.* 1980; 19: 5–12. 7

[6] Hayreh S. S. Ischemic optic neuropathy *Prog Retin Eye Res.* 2009; 28: 34–62. DOI: 10.1016/j.preteyeres.2008.11.002 8

[7] Laties AM. Central retinal artery innervation. Absence of adrenergic innervation to the intraocular branches *Arch. Ophthal.* 1967; 77: 405 - 409. 9

[8] Ye X, Laties AM, Stone RA. Peptidergic innervation of the retinal vasculature and optic nerve head *Invest Ophthalmol Vis Sci.* 1990; 31: 1731 - 1737.

[9] Ehinger Berndt. Adrenergic Nerves to the Eye and to Related Structures in Man and in the Cynomolgus Monkey (Macaca Irus) *Invest. Ophthalmol. Vis. Sci.* 1966; 5: 42–52. 9

[10] May C. A., Lutjen-Drecoll E. Choroidal ganglion cell changes in human glaucomatous eyes *J Glaucoma.* 2004; 13: 389–95. DOI: 10.1097/01.ijg.0000133152.82804.38 9

[11] Lutjen-Drecoll E. Choroidal innervation in primate eyes *Exp Eye Res.* 2006; 82: 357–61. DOI: 10.1016/j.exer.2005.09.015 9

[12] Patterson SW, Starling EH. On the mechanical factors which determine the output of the ventricles. *J Physiol.* 1914; 48: 357–379. 13

[13] Moses R A. Hydrodynamic model eye *Ophthalmologica*. 1963; 146: 137 - 142. DOI: 10.1159/000304511

[14] Fry DL, Thomas LJ, Greenfield JC. Flow in collapsible tubes. DJ Patel, RN Vaishnav. *Basic Hemodynamics and Its Role in Disease Processes*. Baltimore: University Park Press; 1980: 407 - 424.

[15] Maepea O. Pressures in the anterior ciliary arteries, choroidal veins and choriocapillaris *Exp. Eye Res.* 1992; 54: 731–736. DOI: 10.1016/0014-4835(92)90028-Q

[16] Glucksberg M R, Dunn R. Direct measurement of retinal microvascular pressures in the live, anesthetized cat *Microvascular Research*. 1993; 45: 158 - 165. DOI: 10.1006/mvre.1993.1015 13

[17] Kiel J W, van Heuven W A J. Ocular Perfusion Pressure and Choroidal Blood Flow in the Rabbit *Invest Ophthalmol Vis Sci*. 1995; 36: 579–585. 13, 16, 36, 40

[18] Grant WM. Tonographic method for measuring the facility and rate of aqueous flow in human eyes *Arch. Ophthalmol*. 1950; 44: 204 - 214. 17

[19] Friedenwald JS. Contribution to the theory and practice of tonometry *Am. J. Ophthalmol*. 1937; 20: 985 - 1024. 17, 22

[20] Barany EH. A mathematical formulation of intraocular pressure as dependent on secretion, ultrafiltration, bulk outflow, and osmotic reabsorption of fluid *Invest Ophthalmol*. 1963; 2: 584 - 590. 17

[21] Kiel JW. Physiology of the intraocular pressure. J Feher. *Pathophysiology of the Eye: Glaucoma*. Budapest: Akademiai Kiado; 1998: 109 - 144. 17, 19

[22] Silver DM, Farrell RA. Validity of Pulsatile Ocular Blood Flow Measurements *Survey of Ophthalmology*. 1994; 38: S72-S80. DOI: 10.1016/0039-6257(94)90049-3 18

[23] Guyton AC, Polizo D, Armstrong GG. Mean circulatory filling pressure measured immediately after cessation of heart pumping *Am J Physiol*. 1954; 179: 261 - 267. 18

[24] Kiel J W. Choroidal Myogenic Autoregulation and Intraocular Pressure *Exp Eye Res*. 1994; 58: 529–544. DOI: 10.1006/exer.1994.1047 18, 20, 21, 41, 42, 44

[25] Bill A, Linder M, Linder J. The protective role of ocular sympathetic vasomotor nerves in acute arterial hypertension *Bibl Anat*. 1977; 16: 30 - 35. 18

[26] Duke-Elder S. The venous pressure of the eye and its relation to the intra-ocular pressure *J. Physiol*. 1926; 61: 409 - 418. 19

[27] Kiel J W. The Effect of Arterial Pressure on the Ocular Pressure-Volume Relationship in the Rabbit *Exp Eye Res.* 1995; 60: 267–278. DOI: 10.1016/S0014-4835(05)80109-5 22

[28] Friedenwald JS. Tonometer Calibration (An Attempt to Remove Discrepancies Found in the 1954 Calibration Scale for Schiotz Tonometers) *Trans. Amer. Acad. of O. & O.* 1955; 108–122. 22

[29] Baylis W.M. On the local reactions of the arterial wall to changes of internal pressure. *J Physiol (London).* 1902; 28: 220 - 231. 23

[30] Hein T. W., Rosa R. H., Yuan Z., Roberts E., Kuo L. Divergent Roles of Nitric Oxide and Rho Kinase in Vasomotor Regulation of Human Retinal Arterioles *Invest Ophthalmol Vis Sci.* 2009; DOI: 10.1167/iovs.09-4391 24

[31] Davis MJ, Sikes PJ. Myogenic responses of isolated arterioles: test for a rate-sensitive mechanism *Am J Physiol.* 1990; 259: H1890-H1900. 25

[32] Falcone J. C., Davis M. J., Meininger G. A. Endothelial independence of myogenic response in isolated skeletal muscle arterioles *Am J Physiol.* 1991; 260: H130–5. 25

[33] Loutzenhiser R., Bidani A., Chilton L. Renal myogenic response: kinetic attributes and physiological role *Circ Res.* 2002; 90: 1316–24. DOI: 10.1161/01.RES.0000024262.11534.18 26

[34] Meininger G. A., Mack C. A., Fehr K. L., Bohlen H. G. Myogenic vasoregulation overrides local metabolic control in resting rat skeletal muscle *Circ Res.* 1987; 60: 861–70. 26, 27

[35] Johnson PC. The myogenic response. D Bohr, A Somlyo, H Sparks, S Geiger. *Handbook of Physiology: The Cardiovascular System.* Bethesda, MD: American Physiological Society; 1980: 409–442. 24, 25, 28

[36] Rubanyi G.M. *Mechanoreception by the vascular wall.* Mount Kisco, NY: Futura Publishing Co; 1993. 25

[37] Wiederhielm C. A., Bouskela E., Heald R., Black L. A method for varying arterial and venous pressures in intact, unanesthetized mammals *Microvasc Res.* 1979; 18: 124–8. DOI: 10.1016/0026-2862(79)90022-0 25

[38] Johnson P. C., Intaglietta M. Contributions of pressure and flow sensitivity to autoregulation in mesenteric arterioles *Am J Physiol.* 1976; 231: 1686–98. 25, 28

[39] Gaskell W.H. On the changes of the blood stream through stimulation of their nerves *J Anat.* 1877; 11: 360 - 404. 25

[40] Granger H. J., Goodman A. H., Granger D. N. Intrinsic metabolic regulation of blood flow, O2 extraction and tissue O2 delivery in dog skeletal muscle *Adv Exp Med Biol.* 1973; 37A: 451–6. 26

[41] Granger HJ, Shepherd AP. Intrinsic Microvascular Control of Tissue Oxygen Delivery *Microvascular Research*. 1973; 5: 49–72. DOI: 10.1016/S0026-2862(73)80006-8 26

[42] Gidday J. M., Esther J. W., Ely S. W., Rubio R., Berne R. M. Time-dependent effects of theophylline on myocardial reactive hyperaemias in the anaesthetized dog *Br J Pharmacol*. 1990; 100: 95–101. 30

[43] Valleau J. D., Granger D. N., Taylor A. E. Effect of solute-coupled volume absorption on oxygen consumption in cat ileum *Am J Physiol*. 1979; 236: E198–203. 31

[44] Kiel J. W., Riedel G. L., Shepherd A. P. Autoregulation of canine gastric mucosal blood flow *Gastroenterology*. 1987; 93: 12–20. 32

[45] Granger HJ, Goodman AH, Granger DN. Role of resistance and exchange vessels in local microvascular control of skeletal muscle oxygenation in the dog *Circ Res*. 1976; 38: 379 - 385. 32

[46] Schretzenmayr A. Über kreislaufregulatorische Vorgänge an den grossen Arterien bei der Muskelarbeit *Pfluegers Arch Ges Physiol*. 1933; 232: 743–748. DOI: 10.1007/BF01754829 27

[47] Lie M., Sejersted O. M., Kiil F. Local regulation of vascular cross section during changes in femoral arterial blood flow in dogs *Circ Res*. 1970; 27: 727–37.

[48] Hilton S. M. A peripheral arterial conducting mechanism underlying dilatation of the femoral artery and concerned in functional vasodilatation in skeletal muscle *J Physiol*. 1959; 149: 93–111.

[49] Holtz J., Forstermann U., Pohl U., Giesler M., Bassenge E. Flow-dependent, endothelium-mediated dilation of epicardial coronary arteries in conscious dogs: effects of cyclooxygenase inhibition *J Cardiovasc Pharmacol*. 1984; 6: 1161–9. DOI: 10.1097/00005344-198411000-00025

[50] Kuo L., Davis M. J., Chilian W. M. Endothelium-dependent, flow-induced dilation of isolated coronary arterioles *Am J Physiol*. 1990; 259: H1063–70. 27, 33

[51] Koller A., Sun D., Kaley G. Role of shear stress and endothelial prostaglandins in flow- and viscosity-induced dilation of arterioles in vitro *Circ Res*. 1993; 72: 1276–84. 27, 33

[52] Stepp D. W., Nishikawa Y., Chilian W. M. Regulation of shear stress in the canine coronary microcirculation *Circulation*. 1999; 100: 1555–61. 27

[53] Figueroa X. F., Duling B. R. Gap junctions in the control of vascular function *Antioxid Redox Signal*. 2009; 11: 251–66. DOI: 10.1089/ars.2008.2117 28

[54] Segal S. S., Duling B. R. Flow control among microvessels coordinated by intercellular conduction *Science*. 1986; 234: 868–70. DOI: 10.1126/science.3775368 28, 34

[55] Dora K. A., Xia J., Duling B. R. Endothelial cell signaling during conducted vasomotor responses *Am J Physiol Heart Circ Physiol*. 2003; 285: H119–26. 28, 34

[56] Geijer C, Bill A. Effects of raised intraocular pressure on retinal, prelaminar, laminar, and retrolaminar optic nerve blood flow in monkeys *Invest Ophthalmol Vis Sci*. 1979; 18: 1030–1042. 29, 35

[57] Weinstein J. M., Duckrow R. B., Beard D., Brennan R. W. Regional optic nerve blood flow and its autoregulation *Invest Ophthalmol Vis Sci*. 1983; 24: 1559–65.

[58] Shonat R. D., Wilson D. F., Riva C. E., Cranstoun S. D. Effect of acute increases in intraocular pressure on intravascular optic nerve head oxygen tension in cats *Invest Ophthalmol Vis Sci*. 1992; 33: 3174–80. 35

[59] Liang Y., Downs J. C., Fortune B., et al. Impact of systemic blood pressure on the relationship between intraocular pressure and blood flow in the optic nerve head of nonhuman primates *Invest Ophthalmol Vis Sci*. 2009; 50: 2154–60. DOI: 10.1167/iovs.08-2882 29, 37

[60] Riva C. E., Logean E., Falsini B. Visually evoked hemodynamical response and assessment of neurovascular coupling in the optic nerve and retina *Prog Retin Eye Res*. 2005; 24: 183–215. DOI: 10.1016/j.preteyeres.2004.07.002 29

[61] Buerk D. G., Riva C. E., Cranstoun S. D. Frequency and luminance-dependent blood flow and K+ ion changes during flicker stimuli in cat optic nerve head *Invest Ophthalmol Vis Sci*. 1995; 36: 2216–27. 29, 35

[62] Buerk D. G., Riva C. E. Adenosine enhances functional activation of blood flow in cat optic nerve head during photic stimulation independently from nitric oxide *Microvasc Res*. 2002; 64: 254–64. DOI: 10.1006/mvre.2002.2432 29, 35

[63] Riva C. E., Cranstoun S. D., Petrig B. L. Effect of decreased ocular perfusion pressure on blood flow and the flicker-induced flow response in the cat optic nerve head *Microvasc Res*. 1996; 52: 258–69. DOI: 10.1006/mvre.1996.0063 29, 36, 37

[64] Riva C. E., Harino S., Petrig B. L., Shonat R. D. Laser Doppler flowmetry in the optic nerve *Exp Eye Res*. 1992; 55: 499–506. DOI: 10.1016/0014-4835(92)90123-A 29

[65] Riva C. E., Hero M., Titze P., Petrig B. Autoregulation of human optic nerve head blood flow in response to acute changes in ocular perfusion pressure *Graefes Arch Clin Exp Ophthalmol*. 1997; 235: 618–26. DOI: 10.1007/BF00946937 29

[66] Buerk D. G., Riva C. E., Cranstoun S. D. Nitric oxide has a vasodilatory role in cat optic nerve head during flicker stimuli *Microvasc Res*. 1996; 52: 13–26. DOI: 10.1006/mvre.1996.0040 35

[67] Riva CE, Harino S, Petrig BL, Shonat RD. Laser doppler flowmetry in the optic nerve *Exp Eye Research*. 1992; 55: 499 - 506. DOI: 10.1016/0014-4835(92)90123-A 37

[68] Takayama J., Tomidokoro A., Tamaki Y., Araie M. Time course of changes in optic nerve head circulation after acute reduction in intraocular pressure *Invest Ophthalmol Vis Sci*. 2005; 46: 1409–19. DOI: 10.1167/iovs.04-1082 30, 38

[69] Takayama J., Tomidokoro A., Ishii K., et al. Time course of the change in optic nerve head circulation after an acute increase in intraocular pressure *Invest Ophthalmol Vis Sci*. 2003; 44: 3977–85. DOI: 10.1167/iovs.03-0024 30, 38

[70] O'Day D. M., Fish M. B., Aronson S. B., Coon A., Pollycove M. Ocular blood flow measurement by nuclide labeled microspheres *Arch Ophthalmol*. 1971; 86: 205–9. 31

[71] Alm A, Bill A. The oxygen supply to the retina, II. effects of high intraocular pressure of increased arterial carbon dioxide tension on uveal & retinal blood flow in cats *Acta Physiol. Scand*. 1972; 84: 306 - 319. DOI: 10.1111/j.1748-1716.1972.tb05182.x 31, 39, 41, 46

[72] Weiter JJ, Schachar A, Ernest JT. Control of intraocular blood flow. I. Intraocular pressure *Invest Ophthalmol*. 1973; 12: 327–334. 31, 39

[73] Alm A, Bill A. Ocular and optic nerve blood flow at normal and increased intraocular pressures in monkeys (macaca irus): a study with radioactively labeled microspheres including flow determinations in brain and some other tissues *Exp. Eye. Res*. 1973; 15: 15–29. DOI: 10.1016/0014-4835(73)90185-1 31, 39, 46, 51, 53

[74] Kiel J W, Shepherd A P. Autoregulation of Choroidal Blood Flow in the Rabbit *Invest Ophthalmol Vis Sci*. 1992; 33: 2399–2410. 36, 41, 43

[75] Kiel J W. Modulation of choroidal autoregulation in the rabbit. *Exp Eye Res*. 1999; 69: 413–429. DOI: 10.1006/exer.1999.0717 36, 38, 40, 41

[76] Kiel J W, Lovell M O. Adrenergic Modulation of Choroidal Blood Flow in the Rabbit *Invest Ophthalmol Vis Sci*. 1996; 37: 673–679. 38, 40, 56

[77] Kiel J W. Endothelin modulation of choroidal blood flow *Exp Eye Res*. 2000; 71: 543 - 550. DOI: 10.1006/exer.2000.0911 41

[78] Riva C. E., Cranstoun S. D., Mann R. M., Barnes G. E. Local choroidal blood flow in the cat by laser Doppler flowmetry *Invest Ophthalmol Vis Sci*. 1994; 35: 608–18. 41

[79] Wang L., Grant C., Fortune B., Cioffi G. A. Retinal and choroidal vasoreactivity to altered $PaCO_2$ in rat measured with a modified microsphere technique *Exp Eye Res*. 2008; 86: 908–13. DOI: 10.1016/j.exer.2008.03.005 41

Author's Biography

JEFFREY W. KIEL

Jeffrey W. Kiel received his Ph.D. in Physiology from the University of Texas Health Science Center at San Antonio in 1987. His early research focused on gastrointestinal vascular regulation, and then in 1990 he changed directions and began studying the eye. He has worked on choroidal blood flow regulation, the role of ciliary blood flow in aqueous production and, most recently, on the regulation of episcleral venous pressure.